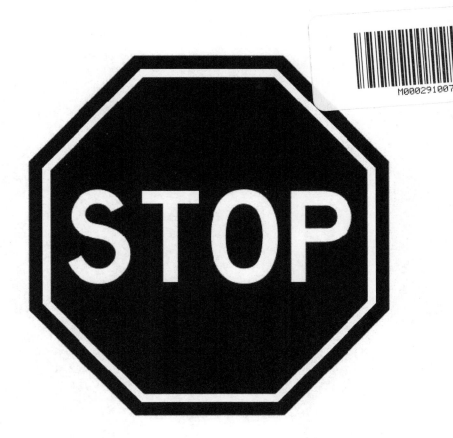
FREE Test Taking Tips DVD Offer

To help us better serve you, we have developed a Test Taking Tips DVD that we would like to give you for FREE. **This DVD covers world-class test taking tips that you can use to be even more successful when you are taking your test.**

All that we ask is that you email us your feedback about your study guide. Please let us know what you thought about it – whether that is good, bad or indifferent.

To get your **FREE Test Taking Tips DVD**, email freedvd@studyguideteam.com with "FREE DVD" in the subject line and the following information in the body of the email:

    a. The title of your study guide.

    b. Your product rating on a scale of 1-5, with 5 being the highest rating.

    c. Your feedback about the study guide. What did you think of it?

    d. Your full name and shipping address to send your free DVD.

If you have any questions or concerns, please don't hesitate to contact us at freedvd@studyguideteam.com.

Thanks again!

CPHQ Study Guide 2019

CPHQ Review & Exam Practice Questions for the Certified Professional in Healthcare Quality Exam

Test Prep Books 2018 & 2019 Team

Table of Contents

Quick Overview

As you draw closer to taking your exam, effective preparation becomes more and more important. Thankfully, you have this study guide to help you get ready. Use this guide to help keep your studying on track and refer to it often.

This study guide contains several key sections that will help you be successful on your exam. The guide contains tips for what you should do the night before and the day of the test. Also included are test-taking tips. Knowing the right information is not always enough. Many well-prepared test takers struggle with exams. These tips will help equip you to accurately read, assess, and answer test questions.

A large part of the guide is devoted to showing you what content to expect on the exam and to helping you better understand that content. Near the end of this guide is a practice test so that you can see how well you have grasped the content. Then, answers explanations are provided so that you can understand why you missed certain questions.

Don't try to cram the night before you take your exam. This is not a wise strategy for a few reasons. First, your retention of the information will be low. Your time would be better used by reviewing information you already know rather than trying to learn a lot of new information. Second, you will likely become stressed as you try to gain large amount of knowledge in a short amount of time. Third, you will be depriving yourself of sleep. So be sure to go to bed at a reasonable time the night before. Being well-rested helps you focus and remain calm.

Be sure to eat a substantial breakfast the morning of the exam. If you are taking the exam in the afternoon, be sure to have a good lunch as well. Being hungry is distracting and can make it difficult to focus. You have hopefully spent lots of time preparing for the exam. Don't let an empty stomach get in the way of success!

When travelling to the testing center, leave earlier than needed. That way, you have a buffer in case you experience any delays. This will help you remain calm and will keep you from missing your appointment time at the testing center.

Be sure to pace yourself during the exam. Don't try to rush through the exam. There is no need to risk performing poorly on the exam just so you can leave the testing center early. Allow yourself to use all of the allotted time if needed.

Remain positive while taking the exam even if you feel like you are performing poorly. Thinking about the content you should have mastered will not help you perform better on the exam.

Once the exam is complete, take some time to relax. Even if you feel that you need to take the exam again, you will be well served by some down time before you begin studying again. It's often easier to convince yourself to study if you know that it will come with a reward!

Test-Taking Strategies

1. Predicting the Answer

When you feel confident in your preparation for a multiple-choice test, try predicting the answer before reading the answer choices. This is especially useful on questions that test objective factual knowledge or that ask you to fill in a blank. By predicting the answer before reading the available choices, you eliminate the possibility that you will be distracted or led astray by an incorrect answer choice. You will feel more confident in your selection if you read the question, predict the answer, and then find your prediction among the answer choices. After using this strategy, be sure to still read all of the answer choices carefully and completely. If you feel unprepared, you should not attempt to predict the answers. This would be a waste of time and an opportunity for your mind to wander in the wrong direction.

2. Reading the Whole Question

Too often, test takers scan a multiple-choice question, recognize a few familiar words, and immediately jump to the answer choices. Test authors are aware of this common impatience, and they will sometimes prey upon it. For instance, a test author might subtly turn the question into a negative, or he or she might redirect the focus of the question right at the end. The only way to avoid falling into these traps is to read the entirety of the question carefully before reading the answer choices.

3. Looking for Wrong Answers

Long and complicated multiple-choice questions can be intimidating. One way to simplify a difficult multiple-choice question is to eliminate all of the answer choices that are clearly wrong. In most sets of answers, there will be at least one selection that can be dismissed right away. If the test is administered on paper, the test taker could draw a line through it to indicate that it may be ignored; otherwise, the test taker will have to perform this operation mentally or on scratch paper. In either case, once the obviously incorrect answers have been eliminated, the remaining choices may be considered. Sometimes identifying the clearly wrong answers will give the test taker some information about the correct answer. For instance, if one of the remaining answer choices is a direct opposite of one of the eliminated answer choices, it may well be the correct answer. The opposite of obviously wrong is obviously right! Of course, this is not always the case. Some answers are obviously incorrect simply because they are irrelevant to the question being asked. Still, identifying and eliminating some incorrect answer choices is a good way to simplify a multiple-choice question.

4. Don't Overanalyze

Anxious test takers often overanalyze questions. When you are nervous, your brain will often run wild causing you to make associations and discover clues that don't actually exist. If you feel that this may be a problem for you, do whatever you can to slow down during the test. Try taking a deep breath or counting to ten. As you read and consider the question, restrict yourself to the particular words used by the author. Avoid thought tangents about what the author *really* meant, or what he or she was *trying* to say. The only things that matter on a multiple-choice test are the words that are actually in the question. You must avoid reading too much into a multiple-choice question, or supposing that the writer meant something other than what he or she wrote.

5. No Need for Panic

It is wise to learn as many strategies as possible before taking a multiple-choice test, but it is likely that you will come across a few questions for which you simply don't know the answer. In this situation, avoid panicking. Because most multiple-choice tests include dozens of questions, the relative value of a single wrong answer is small. Moreover, your failure on one question has no effect on your success elsewhere on the test. As much as possible, you should compartmentalize each question on a multiple-choice test. In other words, you should not allow your feelings about one question to affect your success on the others. When you find a question that you either don't understand or don't know how to answer, just take a deep breath and do your best. Read the entire question slowly and carefully. Try rephrasing the question a couple of different ways. Then, read all of the answer choices carefully. After eliminating obviously wrong answers, make a selection and move on to the next question.

6. Confusing Answer Choices

When working on a difficult multiple-choice question, there may be a tendency to focus on the answer choices that are the easiest to understand. Many people, whether consciously or not, gravitate to the answer choices that require the least concentration, knowledge, and memory. This is a mistake. When you come across an answer choice that is confusing, you need to give it extra attention. A question might be confusing because you do not know the subject matter to which it refers. If this is the case, don't eliminate the answer before you have affirmatively settled on another. When you come across an answer choice of this type, set it aside as you look at the remaining choices. If you can confidently assert that one of the other choices is correct, you can leave the confusing answer aside. Otherwise, you will need to take a moment to try to better understand the confusing answer choice. Rephrasing is one way to tease out the sense of a confusing answer choice.

7. Your First Instinct

Many people struggle with multiple-choice tests because they overthink the questions. If you have studied sufficiently for the test, you should be prepared to trust your first instinct once you have carefully and completely read the question and all of the answer choices. There is a great deal of research suggesting that the mind can come to the correct conclusion very quickly once it has obtained all of the relevant information. At times, it may seem to you as if your intuition is working faster even than your reasoning mind. This may in fact be true. The knowledge you obtain while studying may be retrieved from your subconscious before you have a chance to work out the associations that support it. Verify your instinct by working out the reasons that it should be trusted.

8. Key Words

Many test takers struggle with multiple-choice questions because they have poor reading comprehension skills. Quickly reading and understanding a multiple-choice question requires a mixture of skill and experience. To help with this, try jotting down a few key words and phrases on a piece of scrap paper. Doing this concentrates the process of reading and forces the mind to weigh the relative importance of the question's parts. In selecting words and phrases to write down, the test taker thinks about the question more deeply and carefully. This is especially true for multiple-choice questions that are preceded by a long prompt.

9. Subtle Negatives

One of the oldest tricks in the multiple-choice test writer's book is to subtly reverse the meaning of a question with a word like *not* or *except*. If you are not paying attention to each word in the question, you can easily be led astray by this trick. For instance, a common question format is, "Which of the following is...?" Obviously, if the question instead is, "Which of the following is not....?," then the answer will be quite different. Even worse, the test makers are aware of the potential for this mistake and will include one answer choice that would be correct if the question were not negated or reversed. A test taker who misses the reversal will find what he or she believes to be a correct answer and will be so confident that he or she will fail to reread the question and discover the original error. The only way to avoid this is to practice a wide variety of multiple-choice questions and to pay close attention to each and every word.

10. Reading Every Answer Choice

It may seem obvious, but you should always read every one of the answer choices! Too many test takers fall into the habit of scanning the question and assuming that they understand the question because they recognize a few key words. From there, they pick the first answer choice that answers the question they believe they have read. Test takers who read all of the answer choices might discover that one of the latter answer choices is actually *more* correct. Moreover, reading all of the answer choices can remind you of facts related to the question that can help you arrive at the correct answer. Sometimes, a misstatement or incorrect detail in one of the latter answer choices will trigger your memory of the subject and will enable you to find the right answer. Failing to read all of the answer choices is like not reading all of the items on a restaurant menu: you might miss out on the perfect choice.

11. Spot the Hedges

One of the keys to success on multiple-choice tests is paying close attention to every word. This is never more true than with words like *almost*, *most*, *some*, and *sometimes*. These words are called "hedges", because they indicate that a statement is not totally true or not true in every place and time. An absolute statement will contain no hedges, but in many subjects, like literature and history, the answers are not always straightforward or absolute. There are always exceptions to the rules in these subjects. For this reason, you should favor those multiple-choice questions that contain hedging language. The presence of qualifying words indicates that the author is taking special care with his or her words, which is certainly important when composing the right answer. After all, there are many ways to be wrong, but there is only one way to be right! For this reason, it is wise to avoid answers that are absolute when taking a multiple-choice test. An absolute answer is one that says things are either all one way or all another. They often include words like *every*, *always*, *best*, and *never*. If you are taking a multiple-choice test in a subject that doesn't lend itself to absolute answers, be on your guard if you see any of these words.

12. Long Answers

In many subject areas, the answers are not simple. As already mentioned, the right answer often requires hedges. Another common feature of the answers to a complex or subjective question are qualifying clauses, which are groups of words that subtly modify the meaning of the sentence. If the question or answer choice describes a rule to which there are exceptions or the subject matter is complicated, ambiguous, or confusing, the correct answer will require many words in order to be expressed clearly and accurately. In essence, you should not be deterred by answer choices that seem excessively long. Oftentimes, the author of the text will not be able to write the correct answer without offering some qualifications and modifications. Your job is to read the answer choices thoroughly and completely and to select the one that most accurately and precisely answers the question.

13. Restating to Understand

Sometimes, a question on a multiple-choice test is difficult not because of what it asks but because of how it is written. If this is the case, restate the question or answer choice in different words. This process serves a couple of important purposes. First, it forces you to concentrate on the core of the question. In order to rephrase the question accurately, you have to understand it well. Rephrasing the question will concentrate your mind on the key words and ideas. Second, it will present the information to your mind in a fresh way. This process may trigger your memory and render some useful scrap of information picked up while studying.

14. True Statements

Sometimes an answer choice will be true in itself, but it does not answer the question. This is one of the main reasons why it is essential to read the question carefully and completely before proceeding to the answer choices. Too often, test takers skip ahead to the answer choices and look for true statements. Having found one of these, they are content to select it without reference to the question above. Obviously, this provides an easy way for test makers to play tricks. The savvy test taker will always read the entire question before turning to the answer choices. Then, having settled on a correct answer choice, he or she will refer to the original question and ensure that the selected answer is relevant. The mistake of choosing a correct-but-irrelevant answer choice is especially common on questions related to specific pieces of objective knowledge, like historical or scientific facts. A prepared test taker will have a wealth of factual knowledge at his or her disposal, and should not be careless in its application.

15. No Patterns

One of the more dangerous ideas that circulates about multiple-choice tests is that the correct answers tend to fall into patterns. These erroneous ideas range from a belief that B and C are the most common right answers, to the idea that an unprepared test-taker should answer "A-B-A-C-A-D-A-B-A." It cannot be emphasized enough that pattern-seeking of this type is exactly the WRONG way to approach a multiple-choice test. To begin with, it is highly unlikely that the test maker will plot the correct answers according to some predetermined pattern. The questions are scrambled and delivered in a random order. Furthermore, even if the test maker was following a pattern in the assignation of correct answers, there is no reason why the test taker would know which pattern he or she was using. Any attempt to discern a pattern in the answer choices is a waste of time and a distraction from the real work of taking the test. A test taker would be much better served by extra preparation before the test than by reliance on a pattern in the answers.

FREE DVD OFFER

Don't forget that doing well on your exam includes both understanding the test content and understanding how to use what you know to do well on the test. We offer a completely FREE Test Taking Tips DVD that covers world class test taking tips that you can use to be even more successful when you are taking your test.

All that we ask is that you email us your feedback about your study guide. To get your **FREE Test Taking Tips DVD**, email freedvd@studyguideteam.com with "FREE DVD" in the subject line and the following information in the body of the email:

- The title of your study guide.
- Your product rating on a scale of 1-5, with 5 being the highest rating.
- Your feedback about the study guide. What did you think of it?
- Your full name and shipping address to send your free DVD.

Introduction to the CPHQ Exam

Function of the Exam

The Certified Professional in Healthcare Quality® (CPHQ) exam is required for all candidates seeking Certified Professional in Healthcare Quality® certification. Earning this certification demonstrates one's competency in healthcare quality, dedication to the profession, and ability to improve outcomes across the care continuum. It also can add to a professional's credibility and can distinguish the professional in the field. The National Association for Healthcare Quality (NAHQ) designed the CPHQ to promote professionalism and excellence in the field of healthcare quality. To date, over 11,000 professionals in healthcare quality have achieved certification.

The tasks and objectives defined on the CPHQ content outline are designed based on a job analysis conducted every three years. This job analysis examines the practice and skills of professionals in healthcare quality. Professionals in healthcare quality are defined as those who have on-the-job experience in conducting and/or managing healthcare quality activities such as performance and process improvement, coordination of care, risk management, patient safety, population health, the analysis and measurement of data, performance and quality improvement, and compliance with healthcare regulations. Healthcare quality professionals use administrative, information management, and evaluation skills while performing one or multiple of these functions.

After the job analysis was conducted, those tasks deemed significant to healthcare practice along the care continuum, including acute care, long-term care, home health care, managed care, behavioral health, managed care, and other common care settings. It is recommended that candidates have at least two years of direct experience as a healthcare quality professional. However, there are no formal eligibility requirements to sit for the exam.

Test Administration

Candidates can register online or via a paper application for the exam. The exam is offered in a computer-based format at more than 300 PSI/AMP testing locations around the United State. Some international sites are available as well. Test takers can take the exam Monday through Friday. Evening and weekend availability may be offered. A current photo ID is required to gain entrance into the exam center.

Candidates who successfully pass the exam will receive a certificate, identification care, pin, and information about recertification 6-8 weeks after the date of administration. The Certified Professional in Healthcare Quality® credential remains valid from the date the certificate is received in the mail through a period of two years beginning the on January 1 of the calendar year beginning after the exam was passed.

Retakes are permitted for candidates who fail to pass the test, although a new application must be submitted, and test takers must wait 90 days to reapply. No more than three attempts may occur in 365 days, and if a candidate fails after the third attempt, he or she must wait a full year to retest. Candidates with documented disabilities can receive accommodations according to the Americans with Disabilities Act. PSI must be notified of the requested accommodations at the time of application and scheduling at least 45 days prior to the desired appointment date.

Test Format

The CPHQ contains 140 multiple-choice questions, of which, 125 are scored. The remaining 15, which are randomly scattered throughout the exam, are used to gauge their worth for inclusion in future versions. Of the scored questions, approximately 26% are recall questions, which require the test taker to demonstrate his or her knowledge of specific concepts or facts applicable to the field. The majority of the questions, 57%, are application questions, which evaluate the test taker's ability to interpret and apply given information to a posed situation. Lastly, 17% of questions are analysis questions, which require the test taker to problem solve, integrate information, or use his or her judgement regarding one or multiple situations. Test takers are given three hours to complete the exam. The following table provides the domains on the exam and the number of scored questions for each major domain:

Domain	Number of Questions
Organization Leadership	35
Structure and Organization	
Regulatory, Accreditation, and External Recognition	
Education, Training, and Communication	
Health Data Analytics	30
Design and Data Management	
Measurement and Analysis	
Performance and Process Improvement	40
Identifying Opportunities for Improvement	
Implementation and Evaluation	
Patient Safety	20
Assessment and Planning	
Implementation and Evaluation	

Scoring

An unofficial score report with the pass/fail status is available at the testing site upon completion of the exam. Even those candidates who "pass" must wait to use the CPHQ designation until after the certificate and official results are received via mail. Unofficial score reports also include the number of correct answers. Raw scores are scaled based on the difficulty of the question, which enables scores to be compared across different exams.

Organizational Leadership

Structure and Integration

Supporting Organizational Commitment to Quality

It is a well-known fact that when the leadership team functions effectively, performance improves. As the central organizing body of the organization, leadership has an obligation to deliver all of the functions of administration, including:

- Ensuring cohesion
- Defining vision and values
- Creating and executing strategy
- Ensuring alignment
- Engaging stakeholders
- Developing talent
- Managing performance
- Building accountability
- Ensuring succession
- Allocating resources
- Crafting the culture
- Delivering results

The leadership team is the organization's center. The business performance is dependent upon how effective the leadership team is. Each essential system is integrated and aligned, and every stakeholder must be involved. Balance must also be maintained between competence and capability. Consciousness and character must be balanced against profit and purpose. In order to become a healthy, high-performing organization, individual leaders must define and refine key processes and execute them efficiently. Strategic communication must be consistent and deliver the message in a way that results in organization-wide understanding. Leadership must be actively involved in daily conversations and be engaged enough to unite people around a common cause. This reduces uncertainty and keeps people focused. It also leverages the power of leadership decisions in shaping beliefs and behaviors.

Leaders translate vision and strategic direction into goals and objectives. Systems for performance accountability can clarify what is expected of people. Only then can consequences or rewards be aligned with actual performance. The best organizations develop simple processes that are efficient internally while being locally responsive. Where applicable, processes may also need to be globally adaptable. Establishing and optimizing operational performance is a journey that never ends.

Leaders must hire the best people, then help them develop their skills and knowledge. Leaders must also reward their team so the team members feel confident in their work and choose to remain a loyal employee. Organizations need concrete measures that facilitate quality control. They need to have consistent behaviors, and predictable productivity. In order to obtain the desired results, leaders must establish and maintain a measurement system that provides quality processes. Leaders track progress and compare it to the strategic plan. They consistently review the status of operational results through clear key metrics. Strategies are updated regularly in order to ensure that action is driven by current and verified information focused on achieving the vision.

Without a fully functioning and cohesive leadership team, transformation efforts will not succeed. Transformational leadership occurs when leaders, and the followers they inspire, raise each other to higher levels of motivation and honesty. Transformational leaders use four key characteristics—charisma, inspiration, individualized consideration, and intellectual stimulation—to inspire confidence and to encourage employees to visualize a better future. Transformational leaders question the status quo, and coach employees to develop to their full capability. Creativity, persistence, energy, and sensitivity to the needs of others creates the healthcare environment that for quality improvement.

Studies show that individuals working under a charismatic leader have higher performance and higher satisfaction. They also have lower role conflict when compared to employees working under more structured leaders.

The structure of the leadership team is determined by the organizational structure. Mechanistic organizations are those that have highly complex structure. They are extremely formalized and centralized. Employees of mechanistic organizations are encouraged to perform routine tasks and rely heavily on programmed behaviors. Mechanistic organizations are generally slow to respond to the unfamiliar. They provide fewer opportunities for employees to exercise initiative and generally suppress the individual differences expressed by leaders and followers.

On the opposite end of the spectrum, organic organizations have the structure that is appropriate for changing conditions. It is relatively flexible and adaptive, as an entity, with emphasis on lateral, rather than vertical, communication. Organic organizations are more loosely structured, more innovative, and less specialized. They utilize experts and knowledge rather than position authority, and offer loose responsibilities rather than rigid job descriptions. They emphasize exchanging information rather than handing down instructions. Their decentralized decision-making processes, are less standardized and the division of labor is less structured. Organic organizations impose fewer constraints on the activity of members and they encourage the expression of individual behavior. It is believed that charismatic leadership is more likely to emerge and be effective in organic organizations than in mechanistic organizations.

Value-based leadership is an attitude about people, philosophy, and process. Values-based leaders grant authority to their subordinates, and lead by example. They believe in the ideas of liberty, equality, and natural justice. Some characteristics of values-based leadership are respect for followers, integrity, clear thinking, vision, listening, inclusion, and trust. Values-based leadership often produces social change. The needs of the followers are more likely to satisfied, which may ultimately change the beliefs and behavior of the followers. Values-based leadership provides strategic unity and allows independent initiative.

Participating in Organization-Wide Strategic Planning Related to Quality

Each healthcare organization develops a strategic quality plan in order to guide the organization through the process of setting the right quality initiatives. Without a strategic plan, the organization will jump from one temporary fix to another. Each organization must create a team of quality professionals who can be trusted to ensure that quality products and services are delivered to all customers. If the organization has only one person with the responsibility and knowledge of quality, that person will need to create and educate a team of individuals who can take responsibility for the management of quality within their jobs.

The strategic quality planning process consists of two phases: research and strategy. The research phase includes everything necessary to collect and analyze data before the strategic quality planning starts.

The strategy phase incorporates the steps needed to develop the actual plan. Every initiative must be tied to the key business processes and their performance indicators. Without this step, there would be no real impact on the balance sheet.

The first task of the strategic quality planning team is to examine the existing strategic plan. All team members must understand all of the corporate strategies. The quality strategies they develop must align with and support accomplishing corporate goals. During the research phase the team will evaluate all of the quality initiatives that the organization has used in the past, along with those they will use in the present. They will research and evaluate the significance of tools like Kaizen, reengineering, Six Sigma, and project management. They also need to calculate the cost of quality and compare it to their desire to aim for quality awards.

The team will then determine the answers to these questions:

- What initiatives have been used before?
- What was successful or unsuccessful?
- Why were some of initiatives successful and others not?
- What learning will come?
- Will the learning allow us to reduce the things that prevent success?
- Will it increase the factors that created success?

As a result of the thorough analysis, the team will eventually abandon some initiatives and choose others. They may want to revisit unsuccessful initiatives that they decide might have been done incorrectly or at the wrong time.

The quality strategies must address organizational needs but they must also address customer needs. Customer satisfaction results can identify problems and opportunities. The performance of managers, executives and employees can be assessed by reviewing customer satisfaction. The voice of the customer (VOC) can be obtained through customer surveys, interviews, and focus groups. The results of VOC can point out which quality strategies might help drive new product and service development. Service delivery and competitive positioning can also be improved by listening to VOC. Customer satisfaction levels cannot be determined until the customer's expectations and priorities have been stated.

It is also essential to involve employees when developing quality strategies. Employee input can give additional insight into issues, when employees are encouraged to give voice to their challenges, concerns, and good ideas that might not yet be known. It also ensures employee buy-in during the strategic implementation stage, which ties the quality development into action plans that impact employees directly.

Benchmarking is another way for the strategic quality planning team to decide how they can improve their internal quality processes, their products, and structures. When they know what their competitors are doing they can incorporate lessons learned into the development of their own quality strategies. During the strategy stage the team must create their own vision of organizational quality and develop the strategies to achieve it. This may be the most difficult challenge since it is difficult to anticipate the future of healthcare. For this reason, some teams are more comfortable focusing on clear, short-term goals than on long-term visions that could be incorrect. The team must understand both present and future needs so they can align their organization with appropriate quality strategies which will meet their needs. This is why the team needs to understand the customer and employee needs, wants and desires. It is critical to understand this before a vision can be created. Benchmarking gives the team a picture of what the best of the best have done.

Once the team has set their ideal vision, the team needs to develop and/or update their organizational quality policy. This policy must clarify the overall goal, mandate, and objective for quality. The quality policy should be a brief statement that shows the organizational commitment to quality. With this policy, the organization can ensure that all employees are aware of, aligned with, and support the organization's intentions regarding quality management. The team then creates an operational effectiveness plan, starting by developing objectives that will meet each quality strategy. Detailed action plans are then used to detail how the objectives will be carried out.

Aligning Quality and Safety Activities with Strategic Goals

The strategic quality planning process moves the organization from guessing about quality to clear directions, based upon a well-researched quality plan. Every healthcare organization begins with a goal of caring for the sick and encouraging the health of the well. Strategic planning moves the organization onto a specific track that will ensure that the goals are all accomplished. Although healthcare organizations improve the health of their patients as one piece of their mission, strategic planning enables them to develop a well-organized plan built on the stability of the team. It is essential that the organizational mission, vision and align with the goals of nationally recognized standards of care.

The planning team must also ensure that quality and safety activities are in sync with the strategic quality planning process. Strategic and operational goals have to be reviewed by all team members. Aggregated data can then be scrutinized for trends that could become critical success factors. Identified trends are often used to create key performance indicators (KPI), the measurable results that will decide if the goals and objectives the team sets can be obtained.

The Center for Medicare and Medicaid Services (CMS) has taken the lead in the national goal of transforming health care delivery. That goal aims to "meet the person-centered goals of each individual in creating a health care system that fully engages persons and families in the design, delivery and evaluation of care." In 2016, CMS published the National Quality Strategy for Healthcare. The strategy outlined the objectives and outcomes for action to realize six broad, interrelated goals:

- Goal 1: Make care safer by reducing harm caused in the delivery of care.
- Goal 2: Strengthen person and family engagement as partners in their care.
- Goal 3: Promote effective communication and coordination of care.
- Goal 4: Promote effective prevention and treatment of chronic disease.
- Goal 5: Work with communities to promote best practices of healthy living.
- Goal 6: Make care affordable.

There are also four foundational principles intended to guide the actions of CMS toward the six goals. To ensure that healthcare organizations actively address these principles, and CMS vowed to continuously evaluate how the four foundational principles are embedded within each goal. Those foundations are:

1. Eliminate racial and ethnic disparities
2. Strengthen infrastructure and data systems
3. Enable local innovations
4. Foster learning organizations

The National Quality Strategy was further enhanced in 2017 when CMS announced the comprehensive initiative called Meaningful Measures. This initiative identifies high priority areas for quality measurement and improvement that will improve outcomes for patients and families while also reducing burden on clinicians and providers. Meaningful Measures intends to move payment toward value by focusing efforts on the same quality areas, with the following principles for identifying measures that:

- address high impact measure areas that safeguard public health
- are patient-centered and meaningful to patients
- are outcome-based where possible
- fulfill requirements in programs' statutes
- minimize the level of burden for providers
- are a significant opportunity for improvement
- address measure needs for population-based payment through alternative payment models
- aligns across programs and/or with other payers (Medicaid, commercial payers)

The strategic quality planning team must establish and monitor methods to avoid or reduce the mitigating factors associated with all of the listed items, including high-risk procedures and patient-care services. When preventing mistakes, such as during surgery, both the goals and activities must be clearly defined in a strategy known as mistake-proofing. This involves developing the necessary countermeasures to solve any problems before they actually occur. Mistake proofing is designed to prevent issues that are identified in advance as what could possibly go wrong. Steps can then be taken to ensure that they do not go wrong.

The data associated with implementation must be periodically reported to the governing board, in compliance with fiduciary duty-of-care regulations. The fiduciary duty-to-care rule involves assurances that the board members are acting in good faith, in a prudent and reasonable fashion, and making decisions that are in the best interests of the organization. This regulation allows the board time to prepare a prompt response or adjustment to any detected errors or concerns. Once any errors are addressed, the initiatives can be reintroduced and follow-up comparison data are gathered. The organization's ability to adhere to this cyclical evaluation process is the best quality indicator for positive safety outcomes. The chart below shows a few examples of CMS objectives and possible outcomes.

Goal 1: Make care safer by reducing harm caused in the delivery of care.

Objectives	Desired Outcomes
Improve support for a culture of safety	• Improved application of safety practices involve all team members, patients, and families and assure that individuals' voices are heard • Organizations exhibit strong leadership that educates and empowers the workforce to recognize harm and increase reporting of errors and potential errors • Consumers have increased access to understandable health information • Expanded use of evidence-based services and primary care • Disparities in care are eliminated
Reduce inappropriate and unnecessary care	• Healthcare organizations continually assess adverse events in accordance with evidence-based practices • Healthcare cost reductions are attributable to the reduction of unnecessary, duplicative, and inappropriate care • Disparities in care are eliminated
Prevent or minimize harm in all settings	• HACs, Provider Preventable Conditions (PPCs) and health care-associated infections (HAIs) are reduced • Medication error rates are improved • Falls are decreased • Visibility of harm is improved in all settings • Expanded use of evidence-based services and primary care • Person and family access to understandable health information is increased • Disparities in care are eliminated

Engaging Stakeholders to Promote Quality and Safety

Senior leaders recognize that Including stakeholders in all stages of program development can lead to early buy-in and successful program design. Stakeholders will begin to invest in long-term support for the program. Hospitals generally use three main strategies to engage stakeholders: identifying champions, building strong relationships and communicating regularly with stakeholders, and managing the expectations of the program to be developed.

Champions assist with program growth and development and encourage program stability. Program champions are stakeholders who are deeply involved in the program and influential among their peers. Influential program champions can assist program staff with planning and designing the program and give their expertise based on their previous experiences. They are also extremely helpful in promoting the program and ensuring its continuation and sustainability. They also help manage other stakeholders' expectations. Program champions can offer feedback by identifying areas for clarification and by giving input on potential initiatives. Program staff should share preliminary evaluation results with the champions in order to understand how stakeholders might interpret the results.

Ongoing communication encourages stakeholder support. Ongoing communication with stakeholders enables program staff to introduce themselves as the key contact or source for information about the program. Serving as the key contact guarantees that stakeholders receive correct program information. Stakeholders will refer all questions or concerns to the key contact. Once program implementation begins, communicating routinely with stakeholders about program successes, failures, and new plans will help build support for the program. During the planning and designing stages, program staff should involve the provider community in order to gather input on all of the clinical aspects of the program. Clinicians can become champions and serve as ambassadors to their patients.

CMS developed an emergency preparedness checklist for healthcare facilities that has 70 tasks and gives guidance for developing emergency plans. Healthcare facilities are required to have disaster preparedness manuals and protocols that specify the steps to follow in the event of a one of the following:

- Weather emergencies (tornado, hurricane, thunderstorms, etc.)
- Earthquakes and situations with power loss
- Infectious disease outbreaks
- Bomb threats
- Active shooters
- Bioterrorism
- Infection Prevention
- Case management

Community-based organizations work closely with case managers, physicians, and other members of the healthcare team to coordinate care, so it is important to include these organizations in all disaster preparedness planning. Community organizations working at a local level can promote patient empowerment and self-management. These community vendors can provide a variety of services, including support groups or financial assistance.

Providing Consultative Support to the Governing Body and Clinical Staff Regarding Their Roles and Responsibilities

As health care organizations continue to focus on the American Hospital Association's Triple Aim (better care, better health, lower costs) and shift toward value-based contracting, the top priorities are: improving quality and efficiency of health care delivery, providing better patient care, and aligning with partners to share risk and provide services along the continuum of care. Although it is not required that the board accept responsibility for the daily management of the facility, it is imperative that the board maintain the organization within compliance with fiduciary duty-to-care guidelines.

It is essential that the leadership team work closely with the clinical staff regarding their roles and responsibilities. The three most crucial aspects are credentialing, privileging, and quality oversight. All clinical staff are required to meet stringent competency guidelines surrounding the specific competencies for each role. Credentialing includes allowing a licensed or certified medical professional to provide care within his or her scope of practice. Privileging includes an evaluation of the practitioner's actual performance and qualifications. In healthcare, for a particular provider to become eligible for reimbursement, they must meet a specific set of requirements regarding their educational preparation, clinical experience, and competence. The leadership team must maintain strict oversight of all medical staff by periodically verifying that each individual is qualified to perform their assigned duties. Privileging functions as an internal quality measure for patients. They can trust that the care they receive care is from providers who have demonstrated excellence in clinical practice set by the medical governing board of the organization.

Risk management is the process of identifying actual (and potential) hazards and developing efficient, cost-effective plans to prevent them from occurring. A sentinel event is an adverse incident that has led to, or has the potential to lead to, a catastrophic outcome. Sentinel events require an immediate intervention. After any workplace accident or near miss, it is mandatory to complete an incident report. Within this report are the variables that caused or assisted the problem. Individuals involved are interviewed, the scene is examined, and management is notified.

During the root-cause analysis, the risk-management team utilizes the answers found in incident reports and interviews to determine the main cause of the sentinel event. The focus then changes from the problem to the solution and the leadership team collaborates with the risk-management team to dialogue about gaps in procedures, policies, workforce, and/or environment that need to be addressed. The primary objective in this step is to prevent future occurrences of a similar nature, while preserving the factors that did not contribute to the problem. The best changes to implement are feasible, efficient, and cost effective.

Facilitating Development of the Quality Structure

In order to develop quality initiatives, the healthcare organization must designate quality-improvement councils and committees to build the foundation of excellence. The American Health Care Association (AHCA) was established in 2012 in an effort to improve the quality of patient care in post-acute and long-term-care facilities. This initiative focuses on the achievement of favorably measurable outcomes by March 2021 in four specific areas:

- 10% reduction in hospitalizations
- 10% increase in overall customer satisfaction
- 15% increase in functional mobility outcomes
- 10% reduction in the administration of antipsychotic medications

These specific changes will improve the quality of care delivered and positively impact patient experiences. SMART goals are used to tie the safety activities to the strategic planning process. Roundtable discussions with members at each level of the healthcare team often reveal gaps in care that need to be addressed. Conducting quality strategy meetings may lead significant insights that can be used in the quality plan. During brainstorming sessions, council members look for viable options to reduce variations in quality by eliminating unnecessary or wasteful process steps. As an example, a SMART intervention for each safety initiative may involve several options: hourly rounding on every patient by nursing staff; fall precautions based on age, history, and medications; and remote access to the EHR so physicians may readily view status changes. Each committee can be tasked with creating realistic methods to integrate the plan into current processes.

Assisting in Evaluating or Developing Data Management Systems

Providing exceptional medical care to patients requires that protected health information be safeguarded. The Health Information Portability and Accountability Act (HIPAA) of 1996, a federal statute requiring all entities who care for patients to protect their medical records as protected health information. The portability portion focuses on protecting patient rights to maintain health insurance coverage in the event of a loss of, or change in, employment status. The accountability portion of the bill covers how PHI is guarded. Medical records are to be stored so that access is limited, and strict confidentiality is maintained. HIPAA protections cover all documentation that could reveal diagnoses, treatments, payments, and any other related medical information. Violations of the HIPAA laws may result in severe financial and legal sanctions on the offending organization. Employees who violate HIPAA laws are generally terminated.

Advances in technology continually inform how personal health information (PHI) is entered, stored, and retrieved. Patients must provide their written consent before release of PHI. Healthcare organizations must make each patient aware of the protections and limitations to their PHI policies whenever possible.

With the advent of the EHR, data management professionals within healthcare realized that they must remain attentive to its advantages and disadvantages. The digitizing of EHRs has led to more efficient recordkeeping and increased compliance with documentation standards. It has allowed multiple user access. The leadership team must ensure the PHI is protected through multiple firewalls and gradations of PHI access. In addition, protocols and policies must be in place to for preventing and detecting security breaches. Accreditation entities also require specific strategies and policies to manage PHI. Any failures in this area are damaging to an audit and could slow or derail accreditation efforts. The leadership team must work continuously to ensure that the healthcare organization remains compliant by guarding all aspects of PHI.

Evaluating and Integrating External Best Practices

Historically, evidence-based practices (EBP) are those that have been proven, over time, to yield the most clinically significant impact on healthcare quality and standards. Strict adherence to EBP promotes commitment and professionalism. Many different organizations contribute to the body of knowledge known as evidence-based practices. The leading agencies responsible for shaping the best-practice body of knowledge include: the Institute for Healthcare Improvement (IHI), the World Health Organization (WHO), the National Quality Forum (NQF), and the Agency for Health Care Research and Quality (AHRQ). Combining their endorsed policies, procedures, and practices, these agencies have developed the structure for improving the quality of patient care around the world.

In 2001, the Institute of Medicine produced their "Quality chasm" report which detailed their major concerns about the differences in quality between current healthcare deficiencies and the ideal. The IHI later released a follow up to that report, denoting the six aims for improvement necessary to bridge the chasm: safety, effectiveness, patient-focused, timeliness, efficiency, and equitability. The goal of this report was to spark conversation around healthcare disparities and encourage momentum toward a culture of quality.

The NQF and AHRQ both endorse the utilization of quality performance measures to evaluate processes, patient experience, outcomes, organizational structure. Both agencies also showed that repeated benchmarking (internal and external) fosters healthy competition that is needed to improve healthcare quality. The WHO implemented global efforts of quality and safety by initiating protocols on a larger scale. The WHO considers the importance of implementing healthcare interventions through a culturally sensitive approach. Since the inception of the Global Initiative for Emergency and Essential Surgical Care (GIEESC) in 2005, over 2,300 members and stakeholders from 140 countries have partnered together to improve access to quality healthcare around the world. This globalized healthcare organization has succeeded in changing the healthcare narrative to include underserved and economically-disadvantaged populations.

The Healthcare Effectiveness Data and Information Set (HEDIS) is a tool used by more than 90% of America's health plans to measure performance on important dimensions of care and service. Altogether, HEDIS consists of 92 measures across 6 care domains. HEDIS makes it possible to compare the performance of health plans around the world. Healthcare leaders understand the significance of using evidence based practice to achieve better health outcomes. When the priority is placed on improving quality outcome measures, patients and all other stakeholders reap the benefits.

Participating in Activities to Identify and Evaluate Innovative Solutions and Practices

Innovation is the process of developing new ideas, methods, or actions that improve upon a predecessor. Innovation in healthcare aims to improve current processes, polices, or standards that are outdated or inefficient in an effort to improve outcomes. Advances in technology advances have changed the ways in that healthcare teams research, retrieve, and spread information. It is necessary to identify current trends that will show where, why, and how to allocate resources. The leadership team must be able to use predictive analytics and move toward innovative solutions. Progress cannot exist without innovation.

Once of the primary responsibilities of the leadership team is to remain informed of the fluctuations in industry standards. Some organizations have created leadership positions in strategy and innovation to boost their opportunities to enhance innovation. Other organizations combine the responsibility for strategy and innovation across the whole leadership team.

Two of the most promising healthcare innovations of this decade include telemedicine and predictive technologies. Telemedicine, or telehealth, has reformed healthcare delivery across the country. Providers can now conduct patient assessments, prescribe medications, and collaborate with other medical professionals remotely, via Skype, telephone, email, and secure chatrooms. Distance health eliminates the constraints of geography and mobility, and allows providers access to increasing numbers of previously underserved populations.

Predictive technologies, like patient analytics and medical informatics, help healthcare organizations remain ahead of the curve. Moving beyond the basic EHR, predictive analytics can create a multilingual medical record system. Although efficient, most systems do not communicate with each other. EHRs at two different offices may have software that cannot communicate with each other. This complicates the process and moves further away from a paperless system. Creating a standardized medical software or multilingual software that translates any data into useable information, is required to create a more cohesive EHR system. Information technologists have started working on these issues. Other future innovations include the use of 3D printers to create prostheses, implantable devices, surgical tools, and instruments.

Leading and Facilitating Change

Organizational leaders must have a specific skill set in order to lead and facilitate change. They need good business judgment, strategic insight, comfort with uncertainty, social intelligence, self-awareness, and people management skills in order to thrive. Change management must be a core competency because embracing change and taking risks are requirements for healthcare. The most effective method of facilitating change includes a combination of theories and stages of change.

Healthcare leaders need to execute plans, hold people accountable and be comfortable with a rapid pace of change. There are many different theories related to behavioral change and the stages that an individual goes through in order to achieve lasting change. A few of these theories are detailed here.

The Transtheoretical Model focuses on the thinking process a person goes through even before the active process of change begins. This model has 6 stages:

1. *Precontemplation* occurs when a person has not started thinking about change and may be oblivious to any need for change.

2. *Contemplation* happens when a person is still not ready to make change but is beginning to think about it, and may intend to make changes in the foreseeable future.

3. During the *preparation* stage, the person is prepared to make changes in the immediate future and begins to actively get ready to make changes, such as through creating plans and setting goals.

4. *Action* happens when a person makes clear and decisive changes.

5. Maintenance occurs when the changes are sustained, become enduring habits that continue for a significant period of time.

6. *Termination* occurs when the person has overcome both unwanted behaviors and the temptation to return to them.

Lewin's model of change has three distinct stages: unfreeze, change, and refreeze. Just as an ice cube can be melted, remolded, and refrozen, this model theorizes that the same process works with people seeking change. The first stage, *unfreeze*, involves looking at a situation and recognizing the need for change. It is helping people challenge their current attitudes, habits, or behaviors, in order to make a persuasive case for why change is needed. During the next stage, *change,* new methods are sought, examined, and accepted. Finally, during the *refreeze* stage, these new habits and behaviors are solidified.

In Kotter's 8 step change theory, the first step is to *create urgency,* or to make use of a crisis situation in order to emphasize how urgently change is needed. The next step is to *form a coalition*, which is a team of professionals and family members who will work together to support the person making a change. After that it is important to *create a vision and strategy for change*, with goals and objectives, and then *communicate the vision* to all those who are involved in the process. The next step is to identify and *remove obstacles* that might stand in the way of a person achieving the goals they set. The sixth stage is to *create short-term wins* by recognizing and encouraging the small behavioral changes that are achieved. Once these small steps have been acknowledged, it is easy to *build on the change*, turning the small changes into bigger, long-lasting changes. The final step is to *anchor the change*, making the changes a permanent part of life.

As it applies to healthcare management, diffusion can be defined as the passive and unplanned spread of new practices. Dissemination is the active spread of those new practices to a target audience utilizing planned methodologies. Implementation occurs when those practices are adopted and integrated within a healthcare setting. The spread concept refers to the rate at which newly disseminated ideas or innovations are adopted and implemented. Leaders, acting as change agents, must always be prepared to employ these tactics to facilitate the changes necessary to improve the overall quality of care.

The Diffusion of Innovation theory states that innovations in healthcare spread over time, in five distinct and predictable phases: knowledge, persuasion, decision, implementation, and confirmation. Acting as the change agent, leaders must identify the innovators within the organization and appeal to them in the preliminary stages of the new project, providing knowledge about the concept. It is important to focus on the relative advantage, or benefits, of adopting the new idea over the old. Change agents must also consider ways to persuade innovators of the trialability of the concept, or it if can be implemented on a trial basis, without full commitment. It is essential to confirm that the chosen innovators will communicate their decision to implement the new strategy to stakeholders within the organization. As the use of the new concept or technology spreads within the organization, its implementation will phase out previous behaviors in favor of progress.

Participating in Population Health Promotion and Continuum of Care Activities

Organizational leaders in healthcare must work diligently to develop activities which engage in healthcare promotion and the overall continuation of care of the populations they serve. An episode of care (EOC) is defined as all medical services for one individual patient, for a specific medical condition, from the onset of symptoms to the end of the final treatment. Episode-based payments, also referred to as bundled payments or value-based care, were introduced as a payment system in an effort to contain costs. This payment system is a contrast to the traditional fee-for-service system, which involves physicians receiving payment based on the number of patients that they care for, or the number of procedures they order.

A standardized shift handoff can provide a seamless transition between two different medical staff members who are providing care for the same patient. It can provide detailed and crucial information about the patient and the case. It also indicates official responsibility has moved from one provider to another. This provides a clear mechanism for accountability for oversight of specific tasks. All healthcare facilities have their own internal handoff protocol, with formal handoff training for new staff, ongoing training for established staff, verbal handoff protocols, written handoff forms, and consequences for employees who do not meet handoff standards.

External handoffs occur within two separate healthcare entities or during different transitions of care. Unless the two systems involved have similar procedures, external handoffs can be prone to errors. Standardizing a process may occur through a written checklist, a process flowchart, meaningful acronyms, or an audit tool for staff members to follow. Handoff errors can occur when established standard operating procedures are ignored, written poorly, or are too broad for the scope of the procedure. Errors in handoffs can also occur if medical staff are rushed, are unsure of the team members they are working with, or if they receive incorrect information any time during the patient stay.

The CDC defines transitions of care as the movement of a patient from one setting of care to another. Settings of care may include hospitals, ambulatory primary care practices, ambulatory specialty care practices, long-term care facilities, home health, and rehabilitation facilities. Hospital discharge is a complex process and is a time of vulnerability for patients. Transitions increase the risk of adverse events and miscommunication as responsibility changes hands. Safe and effective transfer of responsibility for a patient's medical care relies on effective provider communication and with the patient's understanding of discharge instructions.

Successful transitions require care coordination and logistical planning to reduce the risk of health complications that could lead to readmission, adverse events, an increase in healthcare costs, or a greater length of stay. A successful transition plan includes, at a minimum, scheduling and keeping appointments, effective medication management, and ongoing medication reconciliation.

Communicating Resource Needs to Leadership to Improve Quality

When the leadership change agent identifies the need for specific resources, it is essential that the findings to be communicated to the rest of the leadership team and the Board of Directors. Staffing and technology needs necessary to perform basic medical-related functions are all upper level decisions with a clear policy. Leaders must be effective resource managers in order to align the organizational mission, values, and goals with the needs of the employees and surrounding community. Internal staffing models can leverage the talent pool against the acuity of the workload of any given unit.

The AHRQ has developed a health information technology initiative to bridge the gap between technology and healthcare. Leadership must consider how social media and other technologies have become a part of the patient culture. Creating a social media presence increases the visibility of the health system and offers opportunities to publicize health information on a global scale. Once consent is obtained, health information in the form of emails and text messages can be sent directly to patients. Telemedicine, as discussed earlier, is also a rapidly growing option for patients with mobility issues or those in remote areas that have a difficult time attending in-person visits.

The Health Information Technology for Economic and Clinical Health (HITECH) Act, which was signed into law by President Obama in 2009 as a component of the American Recovery and Reinvest Act of 2009, supports and expedites the adoption of EHR-provided incentives to those providers who adopted the implementation and use of EHR systems through 2015. The HITECH Act increases the accessibility and exchange of protected health information and supports the electronic exchange of health information using EHR information. Under this act, patients or their appointed designees can gain access to their medical charts in an electronic format. This access enables patients to view their medical history and provides an enhanced method for information sharing among providers.

Providers and organizations must report security breaches related to electronic PHI as soon as it occurs or they will face civil and/or criminal penalties. The HITECH Act also calls for physicians and hospitals that have meaningful use attestation to perform a HIPAA security risk assessment. To move between the three stages of meaningful use, providers must demonstrate the ability to function within each of the stages for two years before they can proceed to the next one.

Recognizing Quality Initiatives Impacting Reimbursement

Historically, physicians have received payment based on the number of patients they provide care for. While the typical pay schedule generally consists of medical providers who are rarely paid incentives based on the care that they provide per qualifying health condition, recent changes to the fee-for-service model have been proposed. One of the most controversial forms of reimbursement includes the pay for performance (P4P) method. Although loosely based on quality indicators, the P4P model can also be seen as incentivizing physicians for efficiency, value, or reporting. It is a patient-centered quality-care model that encourages the development of a relationship between the physician and the patient. Patient perceptions of high-quality care then lead to continued collaboration with their provider. The core P4P model involves compensating providers for achieving specific quality standards or reducing healthcare costs. Quality measures typically include: patient engagement, health outcomes, care coordination, and patient satisfaction.

The current physician value-based modifier system (PVM) and the value-based modifier program (VBM) are quality-based initiatives designed to evaluate practitioners and provide payment based on adherence to specified quality indicators and cost-saving methods, rather than volume. While the P4P concept was proposed through the Patient Protection and Affordable Car Act (PPACA) of 2010, it was closely linked to value-based purchasing (VBP). The VBP operates within hospitals, as a function of CMS, providing a financial incentive for reducing the DRG payments for Medicare patients. In recent years, the shift has been toward the VBM concept, with the stipulation that sanctions will be levied against providers who fail to meet standards of practice.

Proponents of quality initiatives suggest that P4P will encourage physicians to focus on quality over quantity regarding the provision of care. Those in support of this proposal believe that physicians will take more time with each patient, which will serve to improve all of the measures simultaneously. Opponents consider the initiatives to be punitive in nature. Arguments against P4P claim that policymakers do not take into account the increasing numbers of the elderly who will require ongoing care. Increasing patient loads without a compensatory rise in the number of attending physicians will result in poor outcomes across all quality measures. Others have reported concerns regarding the logistics of implementing the reporting technology. Overall, legislators, physicians, and healthcare leaders remain divided on P4P as the primary payer system in healthcare.

Regulatory, Accreditation, and External Recognition

Assisting the Organization in Maintaining Awareness of Statutory and Regulatory Requirements

One of the major roles of the healthcare leadership team is to maintain awareness of all statutory and regulatory requirements and to ensure that the organization meets all of the goals. This role is detailed in the strategic quality plan, where key leaders may be listed as process owners or gatekeepers of individual requirements.

In 2016 CMS unveiled the Overall Hospital Quality Star Ratings on its Hospital Compare website. The rating system combines 64 public measures into a single, one-to-five star rating. CMS rated more than 3,000 hospitals on the star scale. Only 102 hospitals received five stars, the highest rating, while 129 hospitals received one star, the lowest rating. The others fell somewhere in between.

CMS recognizes that one of the most important aspects of any safe patient handling program is support from the top down. Studies have shown that top performers score high consistently, even when metrics change, because they've mastered continuous improvement, not just processes. Senior leaders must have a commitment to constant change and improvement, as well as an aligned structure and reporting processes. Other critical success factors include data availability and analysis, performance improvement methodology, and physician and clinician engagement. Leaders lead, but the activity of the hospitals and systems doesn't stop with leadership. It's an organization-wide commitment to improvement, and it requires a fairly complex and aligned architecture to be functional. It must be systematic, cyclical, and reproducible.

Star ratings may impact the way hospitals are perceived locally and nationally. They allow consumers to easily understand the quality of care like never before. Now patients have a convenient and data-backed rating at their disposal that resembles the same interfaces they experience on other websites. Stars can impact financial value. Current value based purchasing incentives, as well as penalties, are based upon the same metrics that contribute to star ratings. Hospitals and health systems can count on commercial payers taking stock of CMS results, and perhaps having their own proprietary method of comparing provider performance. This is especially applicable in highly competitive markets.

Hospital leaders should foster a high reliability culture where safety is top priority, and several of its high-level corporate goals should relate to safety. When upper management has a commitment to safety transparency the programs are more likely to succeed. At hospitals that have successfully reduced patient handling injuries, it is common to find administrators who support and promote a culture of safety. While weighing the benefits of investing in safe patient handling policies, procedures, training, and equipment, however, hospital administrators may need to fully understand how these investments impact their bottom line. Several case studies by the Occupational Safety and Health Administration (OSHA) have shown that the initial capital investment in programs and equipment needed to safely handle patients can be recovered in two to five years, particularly when equipment purchases are coupled with training and policies to produce a lasting impact. Considerable equipment, training, and infrastructure costs are associated with implementing safe patient handling, but hospitals with successful programs have found that the long-term benefits far outweigh economic costs. Those benefits include:

- reduced injuries
- decreases in lost time and workers' compensation claims
- increased productivity
- higher quality of work life and worker satisfaction
- staff retention
- better patient care and satisfaction

Management support should encompass more than just the workers responsible for direct patient care. Departments such as laundry, maintenance, and engineering are vital to supporting safe patient handling. Management should collaborate with employees and union representatives, where applicable, before launching or expanding a safe patient handling program.

Because there penalties for violating HIPAA are increasing and healthcare organizations obviously want to avoid these penalties, healthcare leaders must develop, adopt, and implement privacy and security policies and procedures. They must also make sure that they are documenting all their policies and procedures, including steps to take when a breach occurs. Leaders should appoint a privacy and security officer who is conversant in all HIPAA regulations and policies.

Healthcare organizations should regularly conduct HIPAA risk assessments to identify vulnerabilities. This will ensure the confidentiality and integrity of protected health information. It is important to remediate any identified risks and revise policies, if necessary, to minimize risk. Healthcare organizations should also adopt policies regarding the use of e-mail. HIPAA does not prohibit the use of email for transmitting protected health information and it does not require that the email be encrypted, but it is best to encrypt email if possible. If an organization can't encrypt email, leaders must make sure that all patients are aware of the risks they are facing if they ask for their health information via email.

Leaders must ensure that their organization adopts strict policies regarding the storage of protected health information on portable electronic devices. They should also regulate the removal of those electronic devices from the premises. HHS has issued guidance regarding the use of mobile devices, and leaders must be familiar with it. All employees who use or disclose protected health information must receive and document their HIPAA training, an essential step to ensuring HIPAA compliance. Healthcare organizations should also conduct refresher courses and train the employees in new policies and procedures.

A notice of privacy practices should be correctly published and distributed to all patients. It should also be displayed on the organization's website, and the organization should obtain acknowledgement of receipt from all their patients. The notice should be updated whenever policies are revised. Healthcare leaders should ensure that they are entering into valid business agreements with all business associates and subcontractors. Any existing business associate agreements must be updated to reflect the changes to HIPAA under the final rule, such as the expansion of liability of business associates. A protocol for investigating potential breaches of protected health information is essential. The risk of harm standard and the risk assessment test can be used to determine if a breach has occurred. If a HIPAA breach has occurred, it is essential that the healthcare organization document the results of the investigation and notify the appropriate authorities. Leaders must implement privacy and security policies, and they should sanction employees who violate them.

The Affordable Care Act was a turning point in U.S. public health policy. Through a series of extensions and revisions, it enforced the multiple laws that together comprise the federal legal framework for the U.S. healthcare system. The Act established the basic legal protections that been absent: a near-universal guarantee of access to affordable health insurance coverage, from birth through retirement. When fully implemented, the Act cut the number of uninsured Americans by more than half, resulting in health insurance coverage for about 94% of the American population, reducing the uninsured by 31 million, and increasing Medicaid enrollment by 15 million.

The first aim of the Affordable Care Act is to achieve near-universal coverage and to do so through shared responsibility among government, individuals, and employers. A second aim is to improve the fairness, quality, and affordability of health insurance coverage. A third aim is to improve healthcare value, quality, and efficiency while reducing wasteful spending and making the healthcare system more accountable to a diverse patient population. A fourth aim is to strengthen primary health-care access while bringing about long-term changes in the availability of primary and preventive health care. The final aim is to make strategic investments in public health, through an expansion of clinical preventive care and community investments.

The Affordable Care Act makes health insurance coverage a legal expectation for U.S. citizens and those who are legally present. The Act created premium and cost-sharing subsidies, established new rules for the health insurance industry, and created a new market for health insurance purchasing. The Act strengthened existing forms of health insurance coverage while building a new, affordable health insurance market for individuals and families who do not have affordable employer coverage or another form of minimum essential coverage. By expanding existing coverage, the Affordable Care Act fundamentally restructured Medicaid to cover all citizens and legal U.S. residents with family incomes less than 133% of the federal poverty level and streamlined

Beyond subsidizing coverage and regulating the insurance and group health plan markets, the Affordable Care Act creates state health insurance exchanges for both individuals and businesses. Exchanges simplify and ease health insurance purchasing by creating a one-stop shopping market for insurance products that qualify for federal tax subsidies and that meet federal and state standards. Under the Affordable Care Act, exchanges are empowered to select qualified health plans, provide information and enrollment assistance, coordinate enrollment with state Medicaid programs, calculate subsidy eligibility, oversee plans, and provide information to the federal government regarding subsidy eligibility and plan performance.

Qualified health benefit plans, whether sold inside or outside exchanges, will have to meet a series of federal requirements including coverage of essential benefits, defined under the Act to include both preventive services as well as a range of benefit classes that reflect a standard employer-sponsored plan. Qualified health plans also will be required to meet federal standards related to provider network and health-care quality. In addition, qualified health benefit plans will be required to make performance information conforming to national quality measurement benchmarks available to patients and consumers.

Beyond insurance, the Affordable Care Act begins the job of realigning the health-care system for long-term changes in health-care quality, the organization and design of health-care practice, and health information transparency. It does so by introducing broad changes into Medicare and Medicaid that empower both the Secretary of the U.S. Department of Health and Human Services (HHS) and state Medicaid programs to test new modes of payment and service delivery, such as medical homes, clinically integrated accountable care organizations, payments for episodes of care, and bundled payments. All of these changes are intended to allow public payers to slowly but forcefully nudge the health-care system into behaving in different ways in terms of how health professionals work in a more clinically integrated fashion, measure the quality of their care and report on their performance, and target for quality improvement serious and chronic health conditions that result in frequent hospital admissions and readmissions.

The Affordable Care Act also invests in the development of a multi-payer National Quality Strategy, whose purpose is to generate multi-payer quality and efficiency measures to promote value purchasing, greater safety, and far more extensive health information across public and private insurers. The Act lays the groundwork for performance reporting on a system-wide basis so that patients can more readily get information about their own health care and how their health-care providers perform. In addition, the Act establishes the Institute for Comparative Clinical Effectiveness Research to promote the type of research essential to identifying the most appropriate and efficient means of delivering health care for diverse patient populations. Throughout these initiatives to improve quality and information, the Affordable Care Act emphasizes efforts to collect information about health and health-care disparities to allow the nation to better assess progress not only for the population as a whole, but also for patient subpopulations who are at elevated risk for poor health outcomes.

The Affordable Care Act provides for the development of a national prevention plan and the establishment of a Prevention and Public Health Trust Fund to finance community investments that will improve public health. The Fund, with a value set at $15 billion, provides additional funding for prevention activities beginning in FY 2010 and continuing annually. The Act also targets Indian healthcare, which received focused attention aimed at improving the performance of health and healthcare programs. New investments are made in school-based health centers, oral healthcare prevention activities, tobacco cessation programs for Medicaid-enrolled pregnant women, and the addition of personalized prevention planning to Medicare.

Identifying Appropriate Accreditation, Certification, and Recognition Options

Once a healthcare organization achieves the status of a certified provider through CMS and OSHA, the next step is to begin developing a plan to identify appropriate accreditation, certification, and recognition options. Potential employees and patients often diligently pursue healthcare organizations with specific certifications and accreditations, as they recognize the brand as a distinction of both quality and excellence. Competitors in the healthcare arena value distinction and recognition, since the standard of care is elevated and therefore signifies advances in clinical practice. Overall, the systematic appraisal of the care provided in hospitals, nursing facilities, and other healthcare organizations serves as a safeguard for patients and ensures that national industry standards are upheld. Continued certification or accreditation over time signifies an ongoing commitment to nationally recognized benchmarks for patient care. Although the CMS and OSHA inspections and subsequent endorsements are mandatory, not every certification, recognition, or accreditation standard is required.

Although often used interchangeably and similar in various ways, the concepts of accreditation and certification are not synonymous. Accreditation is the voluntary process of evaluation of an organization, program, or agency by an impartial third party, resulting in the determination of the presence of the capacity to produce positive outcomes according to a set of nationally recognized standards or practices. One example is laboratory accreditation through The Joint Commission, which ensures that laboratory services are providing superior and accurate results. Certification is also voluntary, and is typically granted to individuals, agencies, facilities, and programs. It is also conducted by a neutral third party and signifies that the recipient has exhibited the ability to provide specialized services. Obtaining the Certification as a Professional in Healthcare Quality shows an outstanding commitment to quality and patient safety.

For the leadership teams of healthcare organizations, one of the most important objectives is to develop a vision of the organization as a whole and to ensure that accreditation is maintained. Certification and accreditation entities have the unique ability to analyze processes and goals and can assist the organization in maintaining accreditation. The accreditation and regulatory bodies provide an unbiased, comprehensive assessment of the attributes of specific clinical programs and services of healthcare organizations. Additional benefits of accreditation and certification include risk management, increased access to funding sources that recognize a specific entity, accountability, process improvement, and business networking opportunities. As a result of the successful completion of the comprehensive assessment, any deficiencies are identified, and excellence is rewarded.

The entire process of achieving recognition is a time-consuming enterprise. Effective leaders have the foresight to consider which types of distinction are crucial in the infancy stage of the development of the organization. While considering the scope of the evaluation, the organization must be prepared to complete an initial self-evaluation. This critical step can identify gaps and redundancies in established processes prior to the site visit. An internal evaluation led by the leadership team can help in the coordination of survey teams, each assigned to streamline processes to meet the rigorous standards of the chosen entity. Policy and procedure manuals must demonstrate the typical lifecycle of a patient receiving care. Process flows depicting the application of current policies and procedures will also be necessary in an effort to confirm authenticity.

There are numerous options for healthcare organizations seeking distinction as excellent service providers. The most notable include the International Organization for Standardization (ISO), National Committee for Quality Assurance (NCQA), The Joint Commission (TJC), Accreditation Association of Ambulatory Healthcare (AAHC), Commission on Accreditation of Rehabilitation Facilities (CARF), Det Norske Veritas & Germanischer Lloyd (DNVGL), Baldrige, and Magnet. Each entity has its own distinct application and survey preparation process, evaluation procedures and duration for its award.

The following table shows certifying agencies:

Entity & Inception year	ISO 1947	NCQA 1990	TJC 1951	AAHC 2010	CARF 1966	DNVGL 2008	Baldrige 1987	Magnet 1983
Certification or Accreditation	Cert	Acc	Both	Acc	Acc	Acc includes ISO	Acc	Cert
On-Site Evaluation	Yes	No	Yes	No	Yes	Yes	No	Yes
Scope of Evaluation	Entire site	Site specific	Entire site	Site specific	Site specific	Entire site	Yes	Yes
Survey process	Yes	No	Yes	Yes	Yes	Yes	Yes	Annual
National Acceptance	Yes global	Yes	Yes	Yes	Yes	Yes global	Yes	Annual
Award Length	3 yrs	2 and 3 yrs by level	3 yrs	3 yrs	1-3	annual	annual	4 yrs

Assisting with Survey of Accreditation Readiness

Excellence in leadership requires a distinct level of expertise in vigilant surveillance. Once the leadership team has established which statutory and regulatory requirements are applicable to the organization, it is essential that the team members thoroughly understand the various standards of the accrediting bodies. Each organization will need to determine which entities provide the types of recognition that they seek and which will be the most valuable to their organization. Conversely, the leadership team must also consider the importance of accreditation in order to remain competitive in the healthcare marketplace. At each stage of growth, different forms of accreditation or certification become necessary. For example, it is mandatory for facilities that receive Medicare and Medicaid funds to obtain TJC accreditation to become eligible to care for those patients, but Magnet status is only established after several years of practice.

The leadership team must also take steps to prepare the facility and staff for the pending evaluation. Developing a culture of safety, customer-focused service, and clinical excellence is imperative. Discussing the purpose of the accreditation that the organization is seeking and how it will not only impact the company but also each department and individual employee, will bolster participation and commitment to succeed. Staff must also be made aware of the random nature of the on-site visit and the expectation that each individual employee be prepared to participate in any aspect of the investigation. It is ideal if the organization begins the preparation for the assessment within a reasonable time frame, in order to allow time to adjust to any changes in established processes and integrate them into the daily tasks of employees. Daily, weekly, and monthly reminders of accreditation standards and principles during staff meetings, in email correspondence, and on the organizational bulletins and screensavers encourages familiarity with site visit objectives. A simple motto to encourage employees to remember the rationale behind the site visit and to guide their preparation is essential.

The next logical step in preparing for an accreditation site visit is to obtain a copy of the applicable standards, associated fees, and an in-depth self-assessment. Each entity typically utilizes an online application process along with supporting software and web-based evaluation tools to guide those preparing for the assessment. The leadership team oversees the accreditation process, so they must carefully research the standards in each domain and compare the requirements to the current policies and procedures of the organization. Organizations seeking accreditation from The Joint Commission must be prepared to review and demonstrate compliance with the National Patient Safety Goals. Top-performing individuals and departments can be recognized for their adherence to established guidelines listed in site-visit materials.

The methodical review of the accreditation standards and comparison to the existing organizational structure must be followed by a mock review. This step moves beyond self-assessment and presents the leadership and employees with intensive, periodic, and impromptu question-and-answer sessions. This type of preparation provides an advantage to the staff and reinforces their understanding of significant principles. Each simulated interview session can build upon its predecessor, increasing the overall score until the leadership team is satisfied with the results. If not required during the initial application process, the next step is to request a date for the actual site visit.

During the on-site assessment, leaders must remain impartial and have a working knowledge of the organizational structure, policies, procedures, and scope of the accreditation standards. After the opening conference, introduction to the leadership team, and discussion, the site surveyors will begin the actual interviews. In the case of a TJC evaluation, the assessors will conduct both individual and systemic tracer sessions. These roundtable discussions are a hallmark of The Joint Commission survey and include the use of an actual patient's journey through the organization from initial contact to exit. Systemic tracer consultations are related to the review of the metrics associate with staff-to-patient ratios, medication administration, appropriate documentation, and National Patient Safety Goals. The assessment then enters the final phase, and the surveyors tour the facility and complete the exit interview with the leadership team. At that time, the surveyors will present their preliminary findings. Soon after the survey is completed, the final conclusions are disclosed to the management team of the organization. Organizations that do not receive any requirements for improvement (RFI) are notified of findings just prior to their public release. If any RFI are received, the facility will need to provide evidence of that the citations have been addressed and corrected through the submission of an evidence of standards compliance report.

Participating in the Process for Evaluating Compliance with Internal and External Requirements

As previously mentioned, the accreditation and certification process is multifaceted and requires significant preparation and buy-in from all members of the organization. The leadership team members must be equipped with the ability to monitor the organization's rate of compliance with evidence-based standards of practice. As the experts in clinical performance, it is imperative that the leadership team develops a method of gathering the data necessary to reflect adherence to the established requirements of the governing body. It is even more important for them to establish a method for data analysis and interpretation. It is through the clarification of the data that obsolete or ineffective procedures and policies can justifiably be transformed. For healthcare organizations in the position of providing clinical bedside care, there is a particular concern regarding medication use, infection rates, service quality, practitioner performance, gaps in expected outcomes for patients, and reportable events.

<u>Clinical Practice Guidelines and Pathways</u>
When preparing for an on-site evaluation for accreditation, the medication administration policies and procedures of any healthcare organization are crucial. The leadership team, which includes physicians and the chief nursing officer, has the responsibility of deciding which clinical practice guidelines the

organization will follow. When managing the care of patients the safe administration of those medications is of paramount importance. Each clinician bears the responsibility of adhering to the five rights of medication administration, which ensures that each encounter involves: the right drug, the right dose, via the right route, at the right time, to the right patient.

With the advent of EHR, many healthcare facilities have charting at the bedside. This step is thought to encourage the clinician to confirm that all five objectives are met with the additional act of the bedside checks. The nurse is encouraged to review the medications as shown in the EHR, ensure that the EHR and medication taken from the medication cart or Pyxis match, and confirm that the EHR matches the medication retrieved from the med cart and is placed into the correct patient's medication basin. The data are gathered through the nurse actually scanning each medication and clicking the EHR in the appropriate section. In some cases, failure to perform this added task can prevent the administration of the medication and flag the patient chart for review.

Although technology has helped decrease medication errors, adverse drug events remain a significant source of harm. Patients in the ICU may be particularly vulnerable to medication errors due to the complex nature of their care. Prior research has shown that medication errors occur more frequently in the ICU and are more likely to cause serious patient harm or death. This clinical practice guideline highlights environmental changes and prevention strategies that can be employed to improve medication safety in the ICU. Following guidelines and pathways results in fewer medication errors, improves quality of care and quality of life, and reduces risk and professional liability.

There are also several guidelines for infection prevention. The CDC guidelines for preventing the spread of infections in healthcare settings is the basic guideline adopted nationwide. There are two tiers of recommended precautions:

- Standard precautions are used for all patient care. They are based on a risk assessment and make use of common sense practices and personal protective equipment use to protect healthcare providers from infection and prevent the spread of infection from patient to patient. Standard precautions makes the assumption that each person may have an infectious disease, so a prudent person would use protection when dealing with body fluids.

- Transmission-based precautions are used in addition to standard precautions and address the method of exposure the patient may have.

  o 1. Use contact precautions for patients with known or suspected infections that represent an increased risk for contact transmission.

  o 2. Use droplet precautions for patients known or suspected to be infected with pathogens transmitted by respiratory droplets that are generated by a patient who is coughing, sneezing, or talking.

  o 3. Use airborne precautions for patients known or suspected to be infected with pathogens transmitted by the airborne route (e.g., tuberculosis, measles, chickenpox, disseminated herpes zoster).

In addition to ensuring that all employees are educated about infection prevention, the leadership team must determine the best method of ensuring that the protocols are carried out. Leaders may oversee changes to infection control policies and processes and receive regular reports from infection prevention committees or teams. Administration generally also has input into who makes the determination of where patients are placed upon admission. It is not enough anymore to randomly assign beds based upon which floor has the most room. Careful attention must be made to avoid patient cross contamination.

Leadership is also responsible for ensuring that the following processes and policies are followed. These are key measures during site visits for all organizations and are often the cause of errors or sentinel events. In order to ensure patient safety each one must be regularly assessed and policies must be reviewed and updated according to organizational policy. The healthcare organization must have policies and procedures that address the following:

- hand hygiene
- use of personal protective equipment
- respiratory hygiene/cough etiquette principles
- appropriate patient placement
- the proper cleaning and handling of patient equipment and instruments
- the proper handling of textiles and laundry
- safe injection practices
- safe sharps handling and disposal
- the steps needed to clean and disinfect the environment

Service Quality

Leaders understand that service quality is one of the most important factors to monitor. It will always be necessary to make sure that all of the applicable quality indicators are met and that service to all patients remains at the highest level. Practitioner performance is directly related to the provider's ability to maintain a standard of excellence in clinical practice and service delivery. It is also imperative that organizational leaders work with departmental team leaders and managers to encourage their direct reports to consider options for credentialing. This is not only vital to the actual employee, but for the team, department, and organization as a whole. One of the best ways to accomplish this task is through ongoing peer reviews. Despite the fact that most managers are aware of the roles that each individual employee is supposed to play on their team, they may not be aware of how that employee interacts with other team members. It may be even more difficult for the manager to accurately assess the untapped strengths of the members of their team. Peer reviews provide colleagues with the opportunity to share constructive feedback about each other in confidence.

An assumption of value-based payment is that quality of care can be easily measured and reported. In reality, however, performance measurement is still evolving. A major challenge is the sheer number of metrics being tracked. Clinicians sometimes complain that all the data collection is busy work and question how some metrics benefit their patients. A 2014 study found that physician practices spend 15.1 hours per week tracking quality metrics for Medicare and other payers and regulators.

Electronic health records are being reconfigured to help ease the burden, but the learning curve has been steep. For many providers, EHRs have only turned paper-based data collection into an electronic exercise. A related issue is that clinical quality is mostly measured via process metrics, which track whether key tasks, such as preventive screenings, occur. Many stakeholders are pushing for more attention to outcomes. As providers take on more financial risk for patient populations under alternative payment models, additional metrics that track the health outcomes of those populations across care sites will be needed.

<u>Documentation</u>

In a highly regulated, high-risk industry like healthcare, compliance is especially important. Healthcare compliance is the process of following rules, regulations, and laws that relate to healthcare practices. Most healthcare compliance issues relate to patient safety, the privacy of patient information, and billing practices. Healthcare organizations are held to strict standards, regulations, and laws from the federal and state levels. Violations of these laws can result in lawsuits, fines, or the loss of licenses.

Changing laws and regulations can make it difficult for organizations to keep up with healthcare compliance. The following are a few of the governing bodies and federal regulations that oversee healthcare compliance:

- The Social Security Act (funding and requirements for Medicare, Medicaid, CHIP, etc.)

- HIPAA and the HITECH Act (protect patient privacy, requiring healthcare organizations to implement measures to keep patient records secure)

- The False Claims Act (makes it illegal to file a false claim for funds from a federal program)

- The Patient Protection and Affordable Care Act (requirements for insurance, Medicaid)

- The Drug Enforcement Administration and the Food and Drug Administration (regulate the creation and distribution of medication) the Office of the Inspector General (protect against fraud)

The Office of Inspector General (OIG) of the Department of Health and Human Services (HHS) continues in its efforts to promote voluntarily developed and implemented compliance programs for the health care industry. In 1998, the OIG issued compliance guideline for healthcare, stating that at a minimum, comprehensive compliance programs should include the following seven elements:

1. The development and distribution of written standards of conduct, as well as written policies and procedures that promote the hospital's commitment to compliance, including adherence to compliance as an element in evaluating managers and employees;

2. The designation of a chief compliance officer and other appropriate bodies, charged with the responsibility of operating and monitoring the compliance program, and who report directly to the CEO and the governing body;

3. The development and implementation of regular, effective education and training programs for all affected employees;

4. The maintenance of a process, such as a hotline, to receive complaints, and the adoption of procedures to protect the anonymity of complainants and to protect whistleblowers from retaliation;

5. The development of a system to respond to allegations of improper/illegal activities and the enforcement of appropriate disciplinary action against employees who have violated internal compliance policies, applicable statutes, regulations or Federal health care program requirements;

6. The use of audits and/or other evaluation techniques to monitor compliance and assist in the reduction of identified problem area; and

7. The investigation and remediation of identified systemic problems and the development of policies addressing the non-employment or retention of sanctioned individuals.

The adoption and implementation of voluntary compliance programs advanced the prevention of fraud, abuse and waste in health care while at the same time furthering the mission of the organization. Compliance efforts are designed to establish a culture within a hospital that promotes prevention, detection and resolution of instances of conduct that do not conform to Federal and State law, private payor health care program requirements, and the hospital's ethical and business policies. In practice, the compliance program should effectively articulate and demonstrate the organization's commitment to the compliance process. Eventually, a compliance program should become part of the fabric of routine hospital operations. Benchmarks that demonstrate implementation and achievements are essential to any effective compliance program.

Ultimately, the executive leadership must put the framework in place to implement an effective compliance program. Organization leaders can set the tone and encourage transparency and ethical behavior. Instilling a culture of accountability that spreads through the organization, helps every staff member understand why compliance is important.

Most facilities use an electronic health record, which enables documentation to include time of observation, time task was performed, what was done, how it was done, and reaction to intervention. Documentation requirements are dictated by facility policy and regulatory guidelines. Two methods are used: charting by exception and comprehensive charting. Charting by exception means that besides recording of vital signs, only abnormal findings are documented. This charting method is somewhat controversial as so much information about the patient is usually left out. It is sometimes argued that this is the safer way to chart, as only what is deviant from normal is noted, and thus, there is less room for documentation errors. The normal is assumed, unless otherwise noted. This method also saves time, as less information needs to be documented, leaving more time for resident care.

Some facilities prefer a comprehensive method of documentation, charting everything about the patient, normal and abnormal, in a very thorough manner. This way, when the chart is reviewed, all details surrounding any event should be present in the medical record.

Practitioner Performance Evaluation
Peer review, by the ethics committees of the credentials and utilization committees, has long been established by organized medicine as a way to scrutinize professional conduct. Peer review is recognized and accepted as a means of promoting professionalism and maintaining trust. The peer review process is intended to balance physicians' right to exercise medical judgment freely with the obligation to do so wisely and temperately.

The American Medical Association (AMA) Code of Medical Ethics states that physicians have mutual obligations to hold one another to the ethical standards of their profession. Fairness is essential in all disciplinary or other hearings where the reputation, professional status, or livelihood of the physician or medical student may be adversely affected. Individually, physicians and medical students who are involved in reviewing the conduct of fellow professionals, medical students, residents or fellows should always adhere to principles of a fair and objective hearing.

Senior leaders are responsible for ensuring that all records are organized and easily accessible by appropriate personnel while still maintaining HIPAA compliance. There must be adequate storage capabilities for all primary source data, updated licenses, peer reviews, etc. There must be policies that detail the collection, monitoring, and evaluation of information and reporting to medical leadership in a timely manner to ensure that all are renewed before they expire. Hospitals have a legal responsibility to verify provider's identity, education, work experience, malpractice history, professional sanctions and license verifications to protect patients from unqualified providers.

Credentialing is the process of obtaining, verifying, and assessing the qualifications of a practitioner to provide care or services in or for a health care organization. Credentials are documented evidence of licensure, education, training, experience, or other qualifications. The process of credentialing is to verify the accuracy and specific data in organizational documents. For physicians, the credentialing agent will request a copy of the National Provider Databank file, and possibly a credit report, criminal provider databank file, and a credit report and criminal background search. They will also perform a primary source verification. This is the process of requesting and receiving verification of the physician's stated credentials from the entity that issued the diploma or certificate. The Affordable Care Act has substantially increased physician credentialing requirements for Medicare and Medicaid enrollment in an effort to reduce fraud and abuse. Insurance plans must meet increased credentialing requirements including periodic re-credentialing and attestation.

Privileging is the process whereby a specific scope and content of a patient care services are authorized for a healthcare practitioner by a health care organization, based on an evaluation of the individual's credentials and performance. A privilege is defined as an advantage, right, or benefit that is not available to everyone; the rights and advantages enjoyed by a relatively small group of people, usually as a result of education and experience. Privileges are specific to services provided at a specific location. Privileges can only be granted by the organization for services that are performed in the environment or organizations location/building.

Gaps in Patient Experience Outcomes

Patient satisfaction is more important than ever as medical costs and insurance premiums rise and consumers find a greater financial risk associated with their own care. Consequently, patients have had to become more personally involved in their healthcare decisions, ensuring firsthand that they receive the most value for their investment.

Patient satisfaction with the healthcare experience has become a top priority for CMS. Every provider and nurse handoff creates the potential for miscommunication and mistakes so it is inevitable that there will be gaps in patient care regarding expected outcomes. It is critical that the leadership team utilize data gleaned from sources such as patient surveys, focus groups, team meetings, grievances, and complaints.

In May 2005, the National Quality Forum (NQF), an organization established to standardize health care quality measurement and reporting, formally endorsed the Hospital Consumer Assessment of Healthcare Providers and Systems (HCAHPS). The NQF endorsement represents the consensus of many health care providers, consumer groups, professional associations, purchasers, federal agencies, and research and quality organizations. The HCAHPS Survey contains 21 patient perspectives on care and patient rating items that encompass nine key topics: communication with doctors and nurses, responsiveness of hospital staff, pain management, communication about medicines, discharge information, cleanliness of the hospital environment, quietness of the hospital environment, and transition of care. The survey also includes four screener questions and seven demographic items, which are used for adjusting the mix of patients across hospitals and for analytical purposes. The survey is 32 questions in length.

The intent of the HCAHPS initiative is to provide a standardized survey instrument and data collection methodology for measuring patients' perspectives on hospital care. While many hospitals have collected information on patient satisfaction, prior to HCAHPS there was no national standard for collecting or publicly reporting patients' perspectives of care information that would enable valid comparisons to be made across all hospitals. In order to make fair comparisons to support consumer choice, it was necessary to introduce a standard measurement approach.

The survey is designed to produce comparable data on the patient's perspective on care that allows objective and meaningful comparisons between hospitals on domains that are important to consumers. Public reporting of the survey results is designed to create incentives for hospitals to improve their quality of care. Public reporting also serves to enhance public accountability in health care by increasing the transparency of the quality of hospital care provided in return for the public investment. With these goals in mind, the HCAHPS project has taken substantial steps to assure that the survey is credible, useful, and practical. This methodology and the information it generates are available to the public.

Identification of Reportable Events for Accreditation and Regulatory Bodies
An adverse event describes harm to a patient as a result of medical care or harm that occurs in a health care setting. A never events refers to a specific list of serious events, such as surgery on the wrong patient, that the National Quality Forum deemed should never occur in a healthcare setting. The Tax Relief and Health Care Act of 2006 mandated that the OIG report to Congress about such events.

Patient safety event reporting systems are a mainstay of efforts to detect patient safety events and quality problems. Incident reporting is frequently used as a general term for all voluntary patient safety event reporting systems, which rely on those involved in events to provide detailed information. Initial reports often come from the frontline personnel directly involved in an event or the actions leading up to it, rather than management or patient safety professionals. Voluntary event reporting is therefore a passive form of surveillance for near misses or unsafe conditions, in contrast to more active methods of surveillance such as direct observation of providers or chart review using trigger tools. The limitations of voluntary event reporting systems have been well documented. Event reports are subject to selection bias due to their voluntary nature. Compared with medical record review and direct observation, event reports capture only a fraction of events and may not reliably identify serious events. The spectrum of reported events is limited, in part due to the fact that physicians generally do not utilize voluntary event reporting systems.

In order to have an effective and active reporting system, Senior leaders must establish a supportive environment for event reporting that protects the privacy of staff who report occurrences. Reports should be received from a broad range of personnel and summaries of reported events must be disseminated in a timely fashion. A structured mechanism must be in place for reviewing reports and developing action plans. While traditional event reporting systems have been paper based, technological enhancements have allowed the development of Web-based systems and systems that can receive information from electronic medical records. Specialized systems have also been developed for specific settings, such as the Intensive Care Unit Safety Reporting System and systems for reporting surgical and anesthesia-related errors. Studies of EHR event reporting systems generally show that medication errors and patient falls are among the most frequently reported events.

A 2016 article contrasted event reporting in health care with event reporting in other high-risk industries such as aviation, pointing out that event reporting systems in healthcare have placed too much emphasis on collecting reports instead of learning from the events that have been reported. Event reporting systems are best used as a way of identifying issues that require further, more detailed investigation. While event reporting utilization can be a marker of a positive safety culture within an organization, organizations should resist the temptation to encourage event reporting without a concrete plan for following up on reported events

Facilitating Communication with Accrediting and Regulatory Bodies

Communication with the accrediting and regulatory entities does not end with the initial evaluation. Maintaining an excellent standard of clinical practice is ongoing and never ending. At each level within the organization, there must be an expectation that the entire organization works toward individual and collective success. Once a specific recognition has been obtained, the organization must remain diligent in maintaining continued compliance. Leaders must be alert for changes in the standards and practices of the governing bodies and accrediting agencies they work with.

When attempting recertification, senior leaders must have current copies of all manuals that dictate the standards associated with specific accrediting bodies. It is also essential to review the previous assessment in order to ensure that all areas where the organization met or exceeded expectations will continue to do so. Areas of deficiency must be reviewed. In areas that were previously deficient, have enough improvements been made? Next, it will be necessary to observe changes in state and federal laws and amendments for necessary policy or procedural changes. Benchmarking must be done to determine if the organization compares well to competitors. This is important when reviewing the scorecard for the individual facility, and for patient outcomes. The scorecard is a way for the public to monitor the status of any healthcare facility. If the competitors are equally accredited and have scored higher on quality indicators, leaders can utilize this information to gauge areas for improvement. It will then be necessary to prepare the organization to repeat the self-assessment, pretraining, and mock-interview process before the recertification process begins.

For the majority of organizations that provide direct patient care, The Joint Commission is the initial choice for accreditation. Once the accreditation is obtained, it is imperative that any failure to adhere to the agreed-upon standards is reported along with corrective measures. For example, any sentinel events involving the universal protocol, National Patient Safety Goals, or the speak-up initiative must be reported directly to The Joint Commission. It is important to note that although voluntary error reporting is a demonstration of best practice, it does not often yield actionable results.

When a sentinel or near-miss event arises within the organization, it must be reported as both an act of good faith and as a standard of evidence-based practice guidelines with The Joint Commission. Concerns can be filed anonymously online, faxed, or sent via US mail. It is vital that as much information as possible is provided so that The Joint Commission can conduct an investigation of the event. One received, the incident will be cross-checked for other reported infractions within the organization in question. The investigation may begin with written notification to the agency or a site visit if the incident is deemed necessary. The personal information of the individual who files the concern can be shared without fear of reprisal, as the information will not be shared with the offending facility. Any resolution will be communicated to the reporting individual but, if there is no jurisdiction on the part of The Joint Commission, the issue may need to be referred to the state's department of health or legal authorities.

Education, Training, and Communication

Designing Performance, Process, and Quality Improvement Training

Despite a busy and fast-paced work environment, leaders at medical facilities must continuously train their employees. Training solidifies the existing skills of each employee and helps them improve in areas where they lack experience. An effective training program spots individual areas of improvement in order to address them properly and allows every staff member to be independently effective when it comes to performing their roles. This builds confidence, improves overall performance, and brings new ideas into the workplace.

Training must include information about personal and patient safety practices. It reinforces consistency in hospital policies when all employees and medical staff are aware of rules and updates for the organization and the healthcare industry in general. It has been reported that the feeling of being poorly educated is one of the reasons why nurses leave. Training keeps employees satisfied, as it leads to collaboration and cooperation among staff members. It makes everyone feel that they are valued and their contributions are acknowledged.

Senior leaders must be able to design or replicate programs that cater to all types of learners, and are customized specifically for the organization. Training programs must be personalized to specifically address the needs of the organization as well as the needs of the individual employee. Ideally, hospital staff, with direct knowledge of training should be consulted when developing a program. Leaders should take advantage of technology by using new methods of teaching, including simulation and just-in-time training. Screensavers and signs throughout the facility can also aid through passive learning.

Leaders must be mindful that each program's effectiveness must also be developed. Training which doesn't improve he employee skills or competency is a waste of hospital funds, human resources, and employee time. Leaders must assess the needs of the employee for a specific training and define the organization's training objectives before anything else is done. Surveys, patient feedback, performance reviews, and observations from team leaders or immediate supervisor can all be used to determine the educational needs of employees. The results of the employee training needs assessment should be used to define the hospital's training objectives. This will help to solidify expectations for employee performance, following the training. Only after they know their objectives and what method will be utilized for training, can they move to the design, creation and implementation of the program.

The hospital must designate an expected training outcome, which can be measured through performance tests and other forms of evaluation for effectiveness. Methods of instruction can be lectures, written materials, SIM labs, JITs, or seminars/workshops. Some training will be short and others will be extended. The location and times should fit easily into the employee workday. A training and development program can only be effective when it is geared to achieve the organizational objectives and helps improve the skills and competencies of the employees.

The leadership team of any healthcare organization tasked with the development of strategies that improve the quality of current processes. It is necessary to eliminate waste, redundancies, and risks while working to expand currently successful strategies. Clinical excellence can only be obtained by developing processes that enhance the quality of healthcare delivery. Models of clinical excellence should be reviewed in order to determine the best model to utilize. When pursuing excellence, it is highly recommended that healthcare organizations steal shamelessly, the best practices of other organizations.

Providing Education and Training on Performance, Process, and Quality Improvement

Healthcare organizations that seek to obtain and maintain accreditation recognize the advantages as well as the disadvantages of the experience. The majority of facilities are prepared to adopt stringent guidelines in favor of being added to the list of other esteemed organizations. The national brand recognition encourages competition in the healthcare marketplace and raises the standard of excellence for healthcare service delivery across the nation. State and federal laws are also built into most standards of accrediting entities.

The principles of both OSHA and CMS heavily influence the regulations developed by industry experts and provide the checks and balances necessary to sustain operational efficiency and processes. A positive review may also result in lower liability-insurance costs for the accredited organization. Since the application process includes a deep dive into procedures, policies, and risk management, unsafe practices may be uncovered that have the potential to prevent future patient harm. Once the final evaluation is published, facilities that meet or exceed industry standards are lauded for their successes.

Disadvantages are inherent in the process once violations become published. Although the offending facility is provided with a preliminary report, they cannot prevent citations from being publicized. Negative reviews not only impact patients' decisions to seek care at a specific organization in the future; previous patients may also consider the publication of poor practices may have resulted in injury and consider retrospective legal action. One negative report, even if later corrected, can cause a facility to lose a once-stellar reputation and projected revenue. Employees and staff may face sanctions from a negative review as well. A failure to meet the expectations of current policies, procedures, or standard requirements could result in organizational restructuring or possible loss of employment.

Knowing these positives and negatives and understanding how employees might react to both, the leadership team must provide the education and training in a way that is non-threatening manner while fostering employee buy-in. There must be a component that explains what benefits the employee will receive from participating in the training. Leaders must incorporate change theory and project management processes into the training also.

To achieve sustainable change, quality improvement initiatives must become a part of the new culture rather than something additional to do. Most organizational change is not maintained because it is not tied into the current culture or it so different than the culture that employees do not embrace it. Threats to sustainability may be identified both at the beginning of a project and when it is ready for implementation.

The National Health Service Sustainability Model is one example of a model that can be used to identify issues that could affect the long-term success of quality improvement projects. Process control and performance boards might be used to communicate improvement results to staff and leadership. Using a written or visual outline of current best practices for a task (standard work), provides a framework for ensuring that changes that have improved patient care are consistently and reliably applied to every patient encounter. Improvement huddles, short, regular meetings among staff to anticipate problems, review performance, and supporting a culture of improvement are also ways to ensure success.

A project may thrive in a supportive context and fail in a different context. The leadership team developing each training must utilize all the tools available to deliver a quality education product. Status review meetings are regularly scheduled events to exchange information about the project. This is one tool that the project manager uses to check in on the project. Typically, the project manager wants to assess the status of each of the following elements during a status meeting:

- Task updates
- Schedule status update (behind or ahead of schedule?)
- Budget status update (under or over budget?)
- Quality/scope status update (maintaining desired scope/quality levels?)
- Current or anticipated issues (changes, risks, resource issues etc.)
- Next steps

Because the project manager should be able to report up-to-date information to the leadership team it is imperative for the project manager to conduct regular status meetings. Project complexity, the number of team members, and the level of information required will all drive the meeting length and frequency.

Effective status meetings not only benefit the project manager by providing timely task updates, but also benefit the entire team by providing a venue for recognizing milestone achievements, sharing information, and bringing problems/issues to the team. Meetings that fail invariably seem to possess similar dysfunctions. They have poorly developed agendas, ill-prepared team members, poor time management during the meeting, ineffective handling of action items, waste time on tangents, and do not get balanced input from team members.

Meeting dysfunctions have significant negative impacts on the progress of the project. While the impacts on schedule, cost, and quality may be obvious, a more subtle impact is the erosion of the project manager's credibility with his or her team. Team members view the project manager as the person responsible for running smooth, relevant, efficient status meetings. When that doesn't happen, often the project manager is deemed to be weak and ineffective

Evaluating Effectiveness of Performance/Quality Improvement Training

The effective evaluation of performance and process training begins with the determination of the most accurate and appropriate method of measuring success. The team may need to may need to return to the data-collection phase if data are unclear. The analysis phase will reveal the data associated to the problems identified in the define stage of this methodology. If it is determined that there are several identified areas for improvement, the leadership team must scrutinize the data to verify the most crucial areas in need of improvement. These key areas will encourage the team to isolate the primary root causes for a deeper dive into analysis.

One of the primary tools utilized in the analysis phase is the Pareto chart. This quality-control tool helps to emphasize the most impactful problems in order to allocate the appropriate amount of resources to rectify the problem. The Pareto diagram is a graphic representation of the data collected to aid in the visualization of the frequency and root causes of deficits associated with the current processes.

Although the data may not actually meet the basic 100% with regard to total distribution, the data will clearly indicate the most significant variables. This display of the results will help to both quantify and qualify the variables. Pareto charts allow the leadership team to focus operations that deliver on, rather than retract from, the value of the services provided. The data gleaned from the Pareto chart can be the foundation of the process-improvement initiative. Once the team is aware of which problems to address, the next step is to develop creative solutions. Through the internal benchmarking exercise, the team can look at departments in-house with similar issues and subsequent successes. Identifying the top performers in similar roles to participate in staff retraining is essential. Colleagues can normalize the new processes and demonstrate their effectiveness.

The competitive benchmarking option suggests looking to organizations with similar concerns that have succeeded in improving their outcomes. This is particularly effective among healthcare organizations that already possess or are seeking to obtain comparable accreditation. This task can be accomplished through reviewing the publicized summary of a competitor on the website of the governing body.

Developing/Providing Survey Preparation Training

The leadership team will devote considerable time to the development and provision of the preparatory survey required for initial and ongoing accreditation. As previously mentioned, one of the most important tasks is to determine which accrediting bodies are vital and which are optional. The leadership team begin by assembling the department leaders, top performers, risk-management staff, and medical governing board. The group must engage in roundtable discussions regarding their impressions of how each department has succeeded in their adherence to the organization's mission, values, and strategic goals. Wherever possible, established data from competing organizations is utilized and compared to current processes. This strategy will help to answer the following questions: Where are we in reference to our articulated organizational mission, core values, and goals? Have current processes led to success or failure toward the realization of the articulated mission, core values, and goals? Which processes need to be changed, eliminated, or added to achieve our business goals? Where do we go from here strategically? How can we get to where we want to go? How can we operationalize our business objectives as a healthcare organization? Do our proposed safety goals and activities align with established industry standards? The answers to these questions will guide the quality assurance team to prepare for the self-assessment required for accreditation.

Initially, the teams gather the basic timelines and presurvey guidelines from each accrediting body. For the majority of governing bodies, the suggested preparatory schedule allows for at least one year of current-process analysis, followed by status updates every three months. The correct standards and manuals must be obtained from each governing body and reviewed for new regulations as well as updates to prior standards. Previous surveys from the organization must also be scrutinized in order to confirm that any deficiencies or areas where policies or procedures failed to meet industry standards can be highlighted. Next, the committee will sift through the data to determine if any new areas within the organization need to obtain accreditation.

The team must initiate the actual self-assessment, with each individual staff member advised of performance expectations and measurement tools. This communicates individual and collective accountability for the survey results. This culture of expected excellence compels clinical staff to raise their performance to meet or exceed the projected outcome. The fundamental objective in these phases is to compare the organization's specified goals and activities to those proposed by the accrediting body.

Effective governance over survey preparation in the third interval prior to the on-site survey, or within approximately four months, involves documentation. Once the mock survey has been conducted, any gaps in services, polices, or processes will be uncovered. Process flows and policies must be updated and deemed legally appropriate. A separate but easily accessible electronic clearinghouse for the legally verified process and procedural documents must be created. There must also be evidence of strict policies regarding the method of approval regarding requests to update or revise documented processes and procedures.

Lead informatics managers must be named, along with their specific areas of expertise within the organization. Those identified leaders must be prepared to answer the questions of the review personnel and locate all documents associated with their respective departments. Actual staff must also be shadowed to prepare for their interactions with review personnel. Finally, within the month preceding the actual on-site survey, it is highly recommended that the organization conduct a second full-scale mock survey.

Disseminating Performance, Process, and Quality Improvement Information Within the Organization

The final task involved in the development of performance, process, and quality standards for the involves the dissemination of the on-site survey findings within the organization. This part of the process is the most critical facet of the maintenance of performance standards. There can be no uniformity in the application of the results of the new and improved processes if there is no dissemination of the results. If staff members are not made aware of the findings of the organizational self-assessment, they cannot be expected to adhere to them.

Once the survey has been completed and the organization has been privately notified of the results, the information is made available to the public. Similar organizations, patients, and even prospective clinical and ancillary staff can readily review the information. The Agency for Healthcare Research and Quality benchmarks for quality indicators remain central to the maintenance of a culture of commitment to quality and safety. This competitive benchmarking allows the organization to closely monitor and compare the progression of proposed changes to the current processes with their competitors subsequent to their separate on-site survey.

Recent changes noted in the 2018 TJC survey process indicate that the decision categories include: accredited, accredited with follow-up survey, preliminary denial of accreditation, and denial of accreditation. All results, favorable or not, must be provided to the organization in an effort to promote transparency, responsibility, and accountability. The leadership team must utilize all of the information contained in the summary to guide the discussions and generate the momentum necessary to maintain any changes to current processes. Follow-up surveys for those that have received a designation other than accredited will typically occur within two months. When preliminary denial requires the organization to provide additional detail, the organization must provide the information within ten working days. If approved, the organization will become accredited. If no progress has been made, the organization may request a formal appeal with the review board to dispute the findings.

It is necessary to include ongoing staff training after the successful completion of the survey process. Without this, continued quality improvement is not sustained. Leadership must do more than simply encourage clinical staff to personally initiate continuing education. In order to remain current on industry standards, employees must be directed to the website of the accrediting entity to complete specific continuing education credit modules.

The Joint Commission is an approved provider of continuing education credits by the majority of professional organizations, including but not limited to: The Accreditation Council for Continuing Medical Education (ACME), Accreditation Council for Pharmacy Education (ACPE), and American Nurses Credentialing Center (ANCC). Clinical leadership should also consider attending the webinars and trainings offered by the accrediting entity. The training modules review pertinent information regarding each standard, along with industry-specific rationales, and are essential for those involved in the survey process.

For organizations able to achieve accredited status through The Joint Commission, the journey is far from over. As previously mentioned, the procurement of accreditation for the entities that garner reimbursement are most valuable for sizable healthcare organizations. This is due to the federally deemed status that accredited organizations enjoy. For example, accomplishing accreditation through an entity with comparable or more stringent requirements, like The Joint Commission, enables a healthcare organization to waive the survey and certification process with CMS while continuing to remain eligible for federal reimbursement. The organization will receive a federal Condition of Participation certificate of compliance, either through governing entities like TJC or state auditors acting on the behalf of CMS. Despite the fact that each accrediting body has its own reaccreditation cycle, it is incumbent upon healthcare organizations to maintain a state of constant readiness.

Leadership must work diligently with clinical managers to encourage all employees to adopt a culture of safety. This can be accomplished internally through the dissemination of monthly risk reports to managers, to be shared during team meetings. Additional options include quarterly safety newsletters, rewards to top performers who exceed safety standards, and surveys regarding questions or concerns about quality.

Practice Questions

1. When preliminary denial of accreditation by TJC requires the organization to provide additional detail, when must the organization provide the information?
    a. Within one month
    b. Within ten working days
    c. Before the end of the current survey
    d. Before the end of the current month

2. What is the basis for The Joint Commission's adoption of the National Patient Safety Goals?
    a. To force healthcare organizations to prevent mistakes during surgical procedures
    b. To institute inflexible patient-safety measures to provide high-quality care
    c. To encourage healthcare organizations to institute high quality standards for patient safety
    d. To capitalize on the fees paid to The Joint Commission or accreditation

3. During strategic planning, what is the main task of the leadership team?
    a. To lead teams
    b. To act as clinical advisors
    c. To develop strategies
    d. To maintain records

4. What is meant by fiduciary duty to care?
    a. Assurance that the board members of a healthcare organization are prudent, acting in good faith, and making decisions in the best interest of the organization
    b. A measure of the fiscal responsibility of the stakeholders within any healthcare organization
    c. Assurance that the board members of a healthcare organization are applying the specific, measurable, accurate, reliable, and timely (SMART) method of goal setting for the organization
    d. A measure of the ability of the CPHQ professional to control the costs of obtaining and maintaining accreditation and/or certification

5. How are credentialing and privileging different?
    a. Credentialing involves the oversight of licensing to medical professionals under their scope of practice; privileging refers to the evaluation of a practitioner's actual performance and qualifications.
    b. Credentialing is typically based on payment for the number of individuals a physician provides care for, whereas privileging is typically based on the quality of care provided.
    c. Privileging involves the oversight of licensing to medical professionals under their scope of practice; credentialing refers to the evaluation of a practitioner's actual performance and qualifications.
    d. Credentialing is the passive and unplanned span of new practices; privileging is the rate at which the new practices are adopted and implemented.

6. What is the leadership team's first action when preparing for a survey by an accreditation agency?
    a. To assemble all of the policy and procedure books
    b. To inform all the staff of the impending survey by email
    c. To engage department leaders, top performers, risk-management staff, and medical governing board in discussions regarding how each department has succeeded in their adherence to the organization's mission, values, and strategic goals.
    d. To begin writing an action plan

7. What are the two major stipulations of the Health Information Portability and Accountability Act of 1996?
    a. To protect the rights of healthcare organizations to deny medical care to indigent patients, and to prevent unnecessary malpractice suits
    b. To protect physicians' rights to provide medical care, and to hold healthcare organizations accountable for how patients' protected health information is utilized
    c. To protect patients against retaliation when reporting malpractice, and to hold healthcare organizations accountable for how patients' protected health information is utilized
    d. To protect patients' rights to maintain health-insurance coverage in the event of job loss, and to hold healthcare organizations accountable for how patients' protected health information is utilized

8. The Institute for Healthcare Improvement reported the six aims necessary to improve the current quality of healthcare as:
    a. safe, effective, problem-focused, timely, efficient, equitable
    b. secure, effective, patient-focused, timely, efficient, equitable
    c. satisfaction, expectancy, problem-focused, timeliness, efficiency, and eagerness
    d. safe, effective, patient-focused, timely, efficient, equitable

9. Innovation in healthcare can best be described as which of the following?
    a. Passively spreading a new process or spreading it in an unplanned fashion
    b. A form of predictive technology that will enhance physicians' ability to provide medical care
    c. Developing a new process, policy, or standard that improves upon the quality outcomes of previous processes
    d. Providing a format to create uniformity of practice across other departments within the organization

10. Which of the following is true of telemedicine?
    a. It is a form of medical care provided remotely by credentialed and licensed healthcare professionals.
    b. It is prohibited by the Health Information Portability and Accountability Act of 1996.
    c. The primary role of the CPHQ professional.
    d. It is required by the Health Information Portability and Accountability Act of 1996.

11. Which of the following is true of competitive benchmarking?
    a. It is not advised by TJC.
    b. It can be done by reviewing the public summary on a competitor's website.
    c. It helps improve internal quality processes.
    d. It is not necessary for accreditation.

12. What is the suggested preparatory schedule for accreditation?
    a. Six months of current-process analysis in advance of survey
    b. One year of current-process analysis prior to survey
    c. At least one year of current-process analysis followed by status updates every three months
    d. It should begin preparing for the next survey immediately this one ends

13. When meetings have dysfunctions, they impact which of the following?
    a. The quality agenda
    b. The cost and team confidence
    c. The project manager's credibility within the team, cost, schedule, and quality
    d. The schedule and cost

14. What do pareto charts allow the leadership team to do?
    a. Focus on operations that deliver on the value of the services provided
    b. Focus on the just-in-time process timeline
    c. View statistics on their dashboard
    d. All of the above

15. Functions of the leadership team include which of the following?
    a. To ensure cohesion, define vision and values, ensure alignment, and deliver results.
    b. To engage stakeholders, develop talent, and manage performance
    c. To build accountability, ensure succession, allocate resources and craft the culture
    d. All of the above

16. What is value-based leadership?
    a. An attitude about people, philosophy, and process
    b. Leading by example rather than manipulation
    c. Integrity, listening, and respect for followers
    d. Clear thinking, inclusion, and respect

17. What are organic organizations?
    I. Those that have a loose structure with more innovation and less specialization
    II. Those that have expertise and knowledge rather than authority of position
    III. Those that have loosely-defined responsibilities rather than rigid job definitions
    IV. Those with fewer constraints on the activity of members, enabling and encouraging the expression of individual behavior by leaders and potential followers
    a. I and IV
    b. III and IV
    c. I, III, and IV
    d. I, II, III, and IV

18. The strategic quality planning process consists of what two phases?
    a. Planning and implementing
    b. Research and implementing
    c. Strategy and implementing
    d. Research and strategy

19. A patient suspected of having TB would be placed under what type of infection control?
   a. Universal precautions
   b. Droplet precautions
   c. Airborne precautions
   d. Contact precautions

20. Which agency mandated that hospitals designate a chief compliance officer to have the responsibility of operating and monitoring the compliance program, and who reports directly to the CEO and the governing body?
   a. TJC
   b. Medicare
   c. CMS
   d. OIG

21. A whistleblower is:
   a. protected from retaliation under the law
   b. an anonymous person who has information of importance
   c. someone who was recently fired from the organization
   d. all of the above

22. What are the primary goals of the OSHA inspection?
   a. To provide a reference for surveyors to specify deficiencies within the organization being evaluated
   b. To protect the safety of patients and/or residents in healthcare organizations
   c. To provide healthcare to individuals that cannot afford health insurance
   d. To protect the safety of the employees of healthcare organizations

23. What is the difference between accreditation and certification?
   a. Accreditation and certification are the same; both are typically granted to individuals, organizations, and facilities.
   b. Accreditation is typically granted to organizations and facilities, whereas certification is typically granted to individuals.
   c. Accreditation is typically based on the total billed for the number individuals a physician provides care for, whereas certification is typically based on the quality of care provided.
   d. Accreditation is typically granted to individuals, whereas certification is typically granted to organizations and facilities.

24. Protected Health Information (PHI) includes which of the following?
   a. Only the patient's EHR
   b. Physician orders
   c. Medical bills
   d. All of the above

25. Public reporting of the survey results is designed to do what?
   a. Create incentives for hospitals to improve their quality of care
   b. Enhance public accountability in health care
   c. Increase the transparency of the quality of hospital care
   d. All of the above

26. Why is it crucial for the leadership team prepare the entire organization for the on-site survey portion of the accreditation process?
    a. To actively observe any gaps in processes, procedures, and policies prior to the actual survey
    b. To provide a provide uniformity of practice across other departments within the organization
    c. To assure that the leadership team is prudent and acting in the best interests of the organization and in good faith
    d. To encourage competition across other departments within the organization

27. Which of the following are true regarding the Hospital Compare site?
    a. It is free on the internet for everyone.
    b. It communicates the CMS scores for every hospital in the U.S.
    c. It posts the scores for healthcare quality measures.
    a. I and II
    b. I and III
    c. II and III
    d. I, II, III

28. Why are peer reviews important for the maintenance of service quality and practitioner performance?
    a. To help achieve and maintain full accreditation or certification
    b. To prevent any legal violations or citations from accrediting bodies
    c. To provide uniformity of practice across other departments within the organization
    d. To allow colleagues to anonymously provide the constructive feedback necessary to guide performance-improvement initiatives

29. Why is it important to identify and report errors to regulatory and accrediting bodies?
    a. To create an atmosphere of patient-centered care within the organization
    b. To maintain ongoing accreditation
    c. To prevent any sanctions or violations for the organization
    d. To identify the appropriate employees to be held accountable

30. What is a sentinel event?
    a. A method showing how 80% of the process efforts occur as a result of 20% of the causes
    b. An unforeseen occurrence that results in harm or death to a patient or group of patients
    c. All of the medical services for one individual patient for a specific medical condition
    d. An action or inaction that may have resulted in a nonlethal injury to a patient

31. Root-cause analysis is used to do which of the following?
    a. Analyze healthcare systems
    b. Prevent incidents from happening again
    c. Respond to OSHA complaints
    d. Investigate patients

32. Every quality management initiative must be tied to what?
    a. The key business processes
    b. The mission and values
    c. How the competitors are doing
    d. Patient care

33. Internal benchmarking can be described as which of the following?
    a. Comparing similar processes to a competitor within the same industry
    b. Comparing equivalent processes within the same organization
    c. Comparing the general concepts of processes in unrelated industries
    d. Comparing similar processes to those in different industries

34. The HCAHPS initiative goal is to provide a standardized survey instrument and data collection methodology for measuring:
    a. the quality of care in hospitals
    b. patient satisfaction
    c. employee satisfaction
    d. patient perceptions of care

35. What are key performance indicators (KPI)?
    a. Goals for change
    b. What employee evaluations are measured against
    c. Measurable data about organizational goals
    d. Attainable goals

Answer Explanations

1. B: If the answers regarding the issues addressed in a preliminary denial are provided by the organization to the TJC within 10 working days, the TJC will grant the accreditation so long as the answers are acceptable.

2. C: The primary goal for The Joint Commission's adoption of the NPSGs is encourage healthcare organizations to institute high quality standards for patient safety. TJC does not force organizations to comply with regulatory standards; federal regulations require adherence for reimbursement for healthcare services.

3. C: During strategic planning, leadership's main task is to create strategies.

4. A: The fiduciary duty-to-care regulation involves assurances that the board members are acting in good faith, in a prudent and reasonable fashion, and making decisions that are in the best interests of the organization. This rule essentially provides the board time to prepare a prompt response or adjust any detected errors or concerns.

5. A: Credentialing involves the oversight of licensing to medical professionals under their scope of practice, while privileging refers to the evaluation of a practitioner's actual performance and qualifications.

6. C: Involving the staff in the discussion is a priority when preparing for a survey by an accreditation agency. Engaging department leaders, top performers, risk-management staff, and medical governing board in discussions regarding how each department has succeeded in their adherence to the organization's mission, values, and strategic goals is one of the best ways to achieve this goal.

7. D: The two major stipulations of the Health Information Portability and Accountability Act of 1996 are to protect patients' rights to maintain health-insurance coverage in the event of job loss, and to hold healthcare organizations accountable for how patients' protected health information is utilized.

8. D: The IHI aims to make healthcare safe, effective, patient-focused, timely, efficient, and equitable.

9. C: Innovation involves developing a new process, policy, or standard that improves upon the quality outcomes of previous processes. Choice *A* refers to diffusion. Choice *D* refers to internal benchmarking.

10. A: Telemedicine is a form of medical care provided remotely by credentialed and licensed healthcare professionals. It has reformed healthcare delivery across the country. Providers can now conduct patient assessments, prescribe medications, and collaborate with other medical professionals remotely, via Skype, telephone, email, and secure chatrooms. This type of distance healthcare eliminates the constraints of geography and mobility, and allows providers access to increasing numbers of previously underserved populations.

11. B: Competitive benchmarking can help reveal how similar organizations solved defects similar to what a given healthcare organization is facing. The comparative analysis can also illuminate how the current processes are outpacing the competitors, which encourages the integration of what works with what does not work well enough. This approach will help the leadership team to deliver on the promise of providing exceptional care. All hospitals have to post their quality information on their websites for the public view.

12. C: The suggested preparatory schedule for accreditation typically involves a year of planning along with close monitoring.

13. C: Dysfunctional meetings impact the project manager's credibility within the team, cost, schedule, and quality.

14. A: Pareto chart tracks key operations over time.

15. D: Leadership teams have many roles. They should strive to ensure cohesion, define vision and values, ensure alignment, and deliver results. They also should engage stakeholders, develop talent, and manage performance. It is also important for them to build accountability, ensure succession, allocate resources and craft the culture.

16. A: Values-based leadership is based on an attitude of the value of people, processes and philosophy.

17. D: Organic organizations are relatively flexible and adaptive and have a loose structure that is appropriate for changing conditions. They emphasize lateral communication and exchanging information rather than the vertical handing down of instructions. Organic organizations tend to be more innovative and less specialized. They utilize experts and knowledge rather than position authority. They offer loose responsibilities rather than rigid job descriptions. Their decentralized decision-making processes, are less standardized and the division of labor is less structured. Organic organizations impose fewer constraints on the activity of members and they encourage the expression of individual behavior.

18. D: The strategic quality planning process consists of research and strategy. The research phase serves a preparatory phase, which involves everything necessary to collect and analyze data before the strategic quality planning starts. The strategy phase incorporates the steps needed to develop the actual plan. Every initiative must be tied to the key business processes and their performance indicators or there would be no real impact on the balance sheet.

19. C: Airborne precautions are used with patients suspected of having TB.

20. D: The OIG mandated that hospitals designate a chief compliance officer to have the responsibility of operating and monitoring the compliance program, and who reports directly to the CEO and the governing body.

21. A: A whistleblower is protected under law.

22. D: This answer is correct because it refers to the primary goal of an OSHA inspection.

23. B: Accreditation is typically granted to organizations and facilities, whereas certification is typically granted to individuals.

24. D: PHI includes all health information that might identify the patient. Everything in the patient's HER, including physician orders and medical bills is part of PHI.

25. C: Transparency is the goal of public reporting of survey results because it can enhance public accountability in health care. Public reporting of the survey results also creates incentives for hospitals to improve their quality of care.

26. A: This is the way to get a close look at everything.

27. D: In 2016 CMS unveiled the Overall Hospital Quality Star Ratings on its Hospital Compare website. The rating system combines 64 public measures into a single, one-to-five star rating. CMS rated more than 3,000 hospitals on the star scale. This website is free to the public.

28. D: It is often necessary for colleagues to provide input regarding the performance of their coworkers to highlight strengths and weaknesses not readily observed by management.

29. A: Choice *A* is the best answer and clearly articulates why error reporting is significant. Choice *B* is incorrect because this is not the most important reason. Choice *C* is incorrect because sanctions are not automatically levied against an organization that reports errors. Choice *D* is incorrect because individual employees are protected against organizational retaliation when reporting errors; reporters remain anonymous.

30. B: A sentinel event is an unforeseen occurrence that results in harm or death to a patient or group of patients. These events require immediate attention.

31. B: Root-cause analysis is a tool used to evaluate patient safety in healthcare organizations. The process identifies the underlying causes of sentinel and near-miss events and helps develop safeguards to prevent the recurrence of the incidents.

32. B: Quality management initiatives should be tied to the mission and values of the organization to achieve sustainable change. Most organizational change is not maintained because it is not tied into the current culture or it so different than the culture that employees do not embrace it. Threats to sustainability may be identified both at the beginning of a project and when it is ready for implementation.

33. A: Internal benchmarking involves measures among similar organizations in the same field.

34. D: The HCAHPS initiative goal is to provide a standardized survey instrument and data collection methodology for measuring patient perceptions of care.

35. C: Key performance indicators are measurable data about organizational goals.

Health Data Analytics

Design and Data Management

Maintaining Confidentiality of Performance/Quality Improvement Records and Reports

Data management is an administrative process that includes acquiring, validating, storing, protecting, and processing required data to ensure the accessibility, reliability, and timeliness of the data for its users. Healthcare organizations use big data to inform business decisions, gain insight into customer needs, healthcare trends, and opportunities for exceeding the expectations of customers.

To understand the huge quantities of data that healthcare organizations gather, analyze, and store, companies turn to data management solutions and platforms. Data management solutions make processing, validation, and other essential functions simpler and less time-intensive. Leading data management platforms allow organizations to leverage big data from all data sources, in real-time, to allow for more effective engagement with customers, and for increased customer lifetime value. Data management software is essential, as healthcare organizations create and consume data at unprecedented rates. Top data management platforms give organizations a 360-degree view of their customers and the complete visibility needed to gain deep, critical insights into consumer behavior that give brands a competitive edge.

While some companies are good at collecting data, they are not managing it well enough to make sense of it. Simply collecting data is not enough; organizations need to understand from the start that data management and data analytics will only be successful when they decide how they will gain value from their raw data. They can then move beyond raw data collection with efficient systems for processing, storing, and validating data, as well as effective analysis strategies. Another challenge for data management occurs when companies categorize data and organize it without considering the answers they hope to receive from the data. Each step of data collection and management must lead toward acquiring the right data and analyzing it in order to get the actionable intelligence necessary for making data-driven business decisions.

Data management best practices result in better analytics; by correctly managing and preparing the data for analytics, companies optimize output. Healthcare organizations should strive to achieve the following data management best practices:

- simplify access to traditional and emerging data
- scrub data to infuse quality into existing business processes
- shape data using flexible manipulation techniques

The EHR is largely a collection of free-form narrative communicated by healthcare delivery. insights, attributes of processes, prognoses, evaluations, and clinical observations are locked up in narrative. Unfortunately, narrative is not conducive to machine learning, data management, and next-generation analytics. It is only through controlled, structured, electronically-legible, and understood terminology that the value of clinical decision support, alerts, clinical rules, and analytics can be realized. Structured terminologies, also referred to as controlled medical vocabularies, provide the semantics of the concepts being conveyed in the electronic health record, and downstream in the data management foundation for analytics. Terminologies provide consistent meaning, promote shared understanding, facilitate communication, and enable comparison and integration of data. They are essential for interoperability among operational information systems, applications such as EHR sharing, and portability. Laboratory information systems also require these services as they process transactions in and out of the application. They need to translate from sending and receiving language sets.

One significant eMeasure standard definition effort is underway. The National Quality Forum's Health Quality Measures Format has the broad charge of recommending how health information technology solutions can provide the data needed for quality measures. The goal is to automate the measurement, feedback, and reporting of comprehensive current and future quality measures, accelerate the use of clinical decision support to improve performance on these measures, and align performance measures with HIT capabilities and limitations. Healthcare analytics are used to identify inefficiencies in care processes, determine opportunities for improvements, and enhance resource implementations. Lack of appropriate infrastructure, poor data integration and privacy issues are barriers toward adoption of analytics in healthcare.

Compliance with an organization-wide privacy policy is of paramount importance. Each individual with the potential to come into contact with protected health information must be advised of the privacy policy. The clinician must act as the gatekeeper, providing the information about any particular client's case to those specifically entitled to the information. In order to maintain the secured control of access to medical records that information exists on a need-to-know basis. The need-to-know rule refers to individuals who must view the client's protected health information for the sole purpose of providing care. These individuals are to have access to the minimum amount of information necessary to perform the task at hand, nothing more. Only the minimum amount of information required to complete the tasks of caring for the patient should ever be released.

Signed, dated, and witnessed informed-consent forms that outline the types of information that can be released must be a mandatory facet of any treatment plan. Paper documents must be stored under lock and key with access only to the healthcare professional and necessary staff. Destruction of paper documents must occur through shredding, or by professionals proficient in document destruction. For electronic files and reports, the clinician must be diligent in the security of their desktop through the use of computer screen locks, shortened time-out locks, or black-out screens whenever the computer is left unattended. Computer access must also be limited. The clinician should consider placing the computer behind locked doors, with passwords that are changed frequently, multiple firewalls, and careful screening of incoming emails and documents to guard against computer viruses.

Whenever possible, electronic transfer of medical information, including emails and faxes, must be sent securely. The most effective process is to verbally confirm that the fax number is correct and stored in a secure location away from those without a need to know. Information to an individual should be limited to those who must have the information to perform their jobs. Any transmission of electronic medical records must contain a basic disclaimer advising the recipient on how to proceed if the documents were received in error, such as:

- This communication contains confidential information.

- If you have received this information in error, please notify the sender immediately by phone and return the original to the address listed on the form.

- Any distribution or reproduction of this transmission by anyone other than the intended party is strictly prohibited.

That verbiage, or something similar to it, should be added to all documents, emails, and other transmitted medical records. The clinician is the gatekeeper, ensuring that only the correct individuals receive the necessary information.

Designing Data Collection Plans

The Institute for Healthcare Improvement (IHI) has a free data collection plan that healthcare organizations are encouraged to use. As stated previously, shamelessly stealing from the best practices of others is considered a best practice in healthcare. Simple data collection planning is a process to ensure that the data collected for performance improvement are useful and reliable, without being unnecessarily costly and time-consuming to obtain. The benefits of simple data collection planning are:

- It helps to ensure that the data gathered contain real information, useful to the improvement effort;

- It prevents errors that commonly occur in the data collection process; and

- It saves time and money that otherwise might be spent on repeated or failed attempts to collect useful data.

The IHI Simple Data Collection Plan

1. Begin your data collection planning by answering these key questions:

- What question do we need to answer—why are we collecting these data?
- What data analysis tools do we envision using to display the data after we have it?
- What type of data do we need in order to construct this tool and answer the question?
- Where in the process can we get this data?
- Who in the process can give us this data?
- How can we collect this data with minimum effort and chance of error?
- What additional data do we need to capture for future analysis, reference, and traceability?

2. Keep the following points in mind when planning for data collection:

- Seek usefulness, not perfection! Remember, data for improvement are different from data for research. Confusing the two can slow down improvement work. We need data that are "good enough" to permit us to take the next step in improving a process. These data are for learning, not judgment.

- Data recording must be easy. Try to build it in to the process under study. Use sampling as part of the plan to collect the data.

- Design the form with the collector's needs in mind.

- Minimize the possibility of errors.

- Provide clear, unambiguous directions.

- Use existing data whenever possible.

3. Develop your plan by answering the following questions:

- Who will collect the data?
- What data will be collected?
- When will the data be collected?
- Where will the data be collected?
- How will the data be collected?

4. When you developed a method to collect the data, test it with a few people who will be collecting the data and incorporate their ideas for improving the data collection plan.

5. Be aware of the cost of collecting the data relative to the benefit gained from having it.

6. Teach all of the data collectors how to collect the data correctly.

7. Record what went wrong during the data collection so that learning can take place.

8. Audit the data as it comes in for accuracy and completeness. Correct errors early.

Measuring Development

Once the mission, goals, and values of a healthcare system have been evaluated, the leadership team creates a project charter. The project charter is specifically defined to serve as a written file that is a roadmap for process improvement. This written agreement usually includes the primary reason for the project, the goal and scope of the project, expected budget, and roles of each member of the team. Measurement is a critical part of testing and implementing changes. Measures tell a team whether the changes they are making actually lead to improvement.

Outcome measures tell the organization how the system impacts the values of patients, their health and wellbeing and shows the impacts on other stakeholders such as payers, employees, or the community. Some outcome measures might be:

- For diabetes: Average hemoglobin A1c level for population of patients with diabetes
- For access: Number of days to 3rd next available appointment
- For critical care: Intensive Care Unit (ICU) percent unadjusted mortality
- For medication systems: Adverse drug events per 1,000 doses

Process measures reflect how the steps in the system perform and show if the team is on track in their efforts to improve. Some examples of process measures are:

- For diabetes: Percentage of patients whose hemoglobin A1c level was measured twice in the past year

- For access: Average daily clinician hours available for appointments

- For critical care: Percent of patients with intentional rounding completed on schedule.

Balancing measures look at a system from different directions and dimensions. They show how changes designed to improve one part of the system are causing new problems in other parts of the system. Examples of balancing measures are:

- For reducing time patients spend on a ventilator after surgery: Make sure reintubation rates are not increasing

- For reducing patients' length of stay in the hospital: Make sure readmission rates are not increasing

The leadership team must decide where to set the thresholds on their goals and objectives. Benchmarking with competitors and national organizations is a good starting point. Literature review for pertinent data will also give clues where the best thresholds need to be set. As an example, numerous studies have been done on C section rates, so when looking at these rates within an organization, a standard threshold limit can be easily determined. Similarly, infection rates, patient satisfaction, and readmission rates are easily located for benchmarking.

<u>Tools & Techniques</u>

As stated earlier there are numerous internet sites where quality tools, plans, processes and guidelines are free to use. Using these tools helps to standardize the quality process and decreases the time spent collecting data. The leadership team is frequently tasked with gathering and compiling health-related data, validating, analyzing, and drawing specific conclusions regarding how to address noted deficiencies. The task at this stage is to select the most appropriate tools for gathering data as well as the tools used to analyze the data once collected.

Data is either quantitative (over time), or qualitative (numbers and totals) then data can be either continuous or discrete. Discrete data have finite values that can be counted. Continuous data have an infinite number of steps, which form a continuum. Some examples of discrete and continuous date include: (Discrete) number of children in a household, number of languages a person speaks, number of people sleeping in stats class; (Continuous) height of children, weight of cars, speed of the train.

Quality professionals have a good working knowledge of the seven basic tools of quality, first emphasized by Kaoru Ishikawa, a professor of engineering at Tokyo University and the father of quality.

The seven indispensable tools are:

1. Cause-and-effect diagram (also called Ishikawa or fishbone chart): Identifies many possible causes for an effect or problem and sorts ideas into useful categories.

Example of a Fishbone Diagram

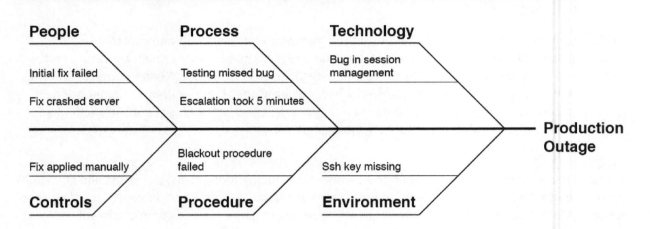

2. Check sheet: A structured, prepared form for collecting and analyzing data; a generic tool that can be adapted for a wide variety of purposes.

3. Control charts: Graphs used to study how a process changes over time. A control chart begins with a time series graph. A central line (X) is added as a visual reference for detecting shifts or trends. This is also referred to as the process location. Upper and lower control limits (UCL and LCL) are computed from available data and placed equidistant from the central line. This is also referred to as process dispersion.

4. Histogram: The graph used most often to show frequency distributions, or how often each different value in a set of data occurs.

5. Pareto chart: Shows on a bar graph which factors are more significant. Also called a distribution diagram.

Example of a Pareto Chart

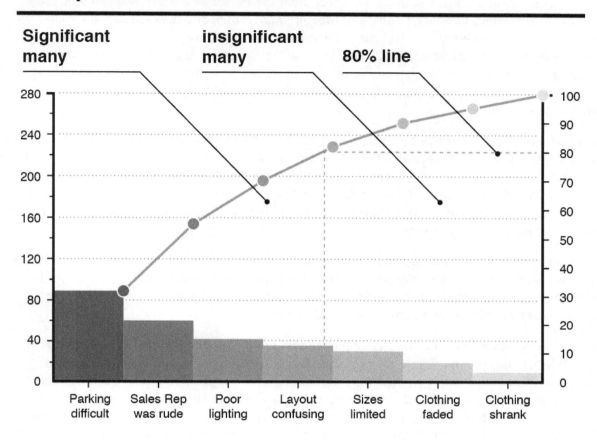

6. Scatter diagram: Graphs pairs of numerical data, one variable on each axis, to look for a relationship.

7. Stratification: A technique that separates data gathered from a variety of sources so that patterns can be seen.

Example of a Stratification

Day	Mon	Tue	Wed	Thu	Fri	Sat	Sun
Frequency - Late in Office	4	2	1	0	0	0	0

In addition to the basic 7, there are numerous other types of quality tools available for use. Free samples of the five why's, Gantt charts, x bar and R charts, z score, and others are all available on quality websites.

Sampling Methodology

Bias is the tendency of a statistic to overestimate or underestimate a parameter. Bias can seep into results for many reasons, including sampling or measurement errors, or unrepresentative samples. Sampling error is the tendency for a statistic not to exactly match the population. Error does not necessarily mean that a mistake was made in your sampling; sampling variability could be a more accurate name. The tendency for statistics to get very close, but not exactly right, is called sampling error. If the statistic is unbiased, the average of all statistics from all samples will average the true population parameter.

Measurement errors occur where a provided response is different from the real value. For example, you might survey to find out if a person voted on a tax increase. A person may have voted for it, but by the way a question is asked, they could be confused by the wording of the questionnaire and mistakenly respond that they did not vote for it. Several factors may cause measurement error, including the way the interviewer poses the question, wording on the questionnaire, the way the data is collected, and the respondent's record-keeping system.

Sampling methods can be classified into two categories. Probability sampling occurs where the sample has a known probability of being selected. In probability sampling it is possible to determine which sampling units belong to which sample and the probability that each sample will be selected. The following sampling methods are examples of probability sampling:

- Simple Random Sampling (SRS): A simple random sample is often mentioned in elementary statistics classes, but it is actually one of the least used techniques. In theory, it is easy to understand. However, in practice it's tough to perform. A random sample is a sample that is chosen randomly. Random samples are used to avoid bias and other unwanted effects. Of course, it isn't quite as simple as it seems: choosing a random sample is not as simple as just picking 100 people from 10,000 people. The random sample must be truly random. To generate random numbers you can open Excel® and follow these steps: Step 1: Type "=RAND()" into an empty cell. Step 2: Press "ENTER." This generates a random number between 0 and 1. Step 3: Click the blue box at the bottom right of the cell to drag the formula up a column or across a row. This generates more random numbers.

- Stratified Sampling: Stratified sampling is possible when it makes sense to partition the population into groups based on a factor that may influence the variable that is being measured. These groups are then called strata. An individual group is called a stratum. With stratified sampling, the population should be partitioned into groups (strata). A random sample should be obtained from each group (stratum). Data is then collected on each sampling unit that was randomly sampled from each stratum. Stratified sampling works best when a heterogeneous population is split into fairly homogeneous groups. Under these conditions, stratification generally produces more precise estimates of the population percents than estimates that would be found from a simple random sample.

- Cluster Sampling: With cluster sampling, the population is divided into groups (clusters). There is a random sample obtained of a certain number of clusters, from all possible clusters. Data is obtained on every sampling unit in each of the randomly selected clusters. It is important to note that, unlike the strata in stratified sampling, the clusters should be microcosms, rather than subsections, of the population. Each cluster should be heterogeneous.

- Systematic Sampling: Systematic sampling is a type of probability sampling method in which sample members from a larger population are selected according to a random starting point and a fixed, periodic interval. This interval, called the sampling interval, is calculated by dividing the population size by the desired sample size. Despite the sample population being selected in advance, systematic sampling is still thought of as being random if the periodic interval is determined beforehand and the starting point is random

- Multistage Sampling: Multi-stage sampling (also known as multi-stage cluster sampling) is a more complex form of cluster sampling which contains two or more stages in sample selection. In multi-stage sampling large clusters of population are divided into smaller clusters in several stages in order to make primary data collection more manageable. It has to be acknowledged that multi-stage sampling is not as effective as true random sampling; however, it addresses certain disadvantages associated with true random sampling such as being overly expensive and time consuming.

- Non-probability Sampling: Non-probability sampling should be avoided because they are volunteer samples and haphazard (convenience) samples, which are based on human choice rather than random selection. Statistical theory cannot explain how they might behave and potential sources of bias are rampant. These are common mistakes and result in sampling disasters.

Projects targeting the improvement of defective processes in healthcare service delivery will require the collection of raw data at various points in the process. Once the project charter has been developed and the appropriate analytical tools have been chosen, the project management team will need to determine how often to collect the data in order to confirm that the appropriate amount of information has been gathered. This step entails asking several fundamental questions. Some of the most crucial include: Where will the data come from? How will we gather the data that we need? What are acceptable intervals within which to collect the necessary data? How will we know when we have what we need?

Participating in Identifying or Selecting Measures

Measures used to assess and compare the quality of health care organizations are classified as either a structure, process, or outcome measure. Structural measures give consumers a sense of a health care provider's capacity, systems, and processes to provide high-quality care. The structural measure generally compares one thing to another. For example, does the health care organization use electronic medical records or medication order entry systems, the number or proportion of board-certified physicians, or the ratio of providers to patients?

Process measures indicate what a provider does to maintain or improve health, either for healthy people or for those diagnosed with a health care condition. These measures typically reflect generally accepted recommendations for clinical practice. For example: the percentage of women receiving mammograms; or the percentage of people with diabetes who had their blood sugar tested and controlled. Process measures inform consumers about medical care they may expect to receive for a given condition or disease, and can contribute toward improving health outcomes. The majority of healthcare quality measures used for public reporting are process measures.

Outcome measures reflect the impact of the healthcare service or intervention on the health status of patients. For example, surgical mortality rates, the rate of surgical complications, or hospital-acquired infections. Outcome measures may seem to represent the gold standard in measuring quality, but an outcome is the result of numerous factors, many beyond providers' control.

Risk-adjustment methods, mathematical models that correct for differing characteristics within a population, such as patient health status, help account for these factors. However, the science of risk adjustment is still evolving. Experts acknowledge that better risk-adjustment methods are needed to minimize the reporting of misleading or even inaccurate information about healthcare quality

Healthcare leaders are always aware of comparative data and benchmarking so they are in the best position to identify and select measures for their organization. High volume processes, error prone processes, safety measures and others that are mandated by CMS or a parent organization can result in an organization monitoring several dozen measures each year

Assisting in Developing Scorecards and Dashboards

A scorecard is a type of report that measures and compares an organization's performance against its projections and goals. Scorecards are sophisticated software solutions; predictive analytics. The scorecard utilizes the organization's data to evaluate the success and failure of key performance indicators (KPIs). Scorecards provide serious value to an organization, if done correctly. With scorecards, businesses can evaluate their goals and direction, determine if they are on track, assess trends and patterns ,and utilize resources in the most efficient way possible.

The scorecard began as a simple performance measurement framework and is now a full strategic planning and management system. It is a framework providing performance measurements of what should be done on a daily basis, measured at every level of the organization. The organizational vision and strategies set by senior management are communicated to every department and level of the organization. Objectives, goals, responsibilities, and accountabilities are set by departments and personnel to align with the vision and strategies. Additional training is included as needed to assist personnel in reaching their goals.

Dashboards typically are limited to show summaries, key trends, comparisons, and exceptions. A good dashboard is simple, has minimum distractions, supports organized business with meaning and useful data, applies human visual perception to visual presentation of information, and enables instantaneous and informed decisions to be made at a glance. Dashboards are made up of multiple reports, allowing leaders to easily compare and contrast different reports or access diverse datasets in one place. Scorecards can be included and viewed on a dashboard with other repository to ensure accuracy within the reports.

Example of a Dashboard

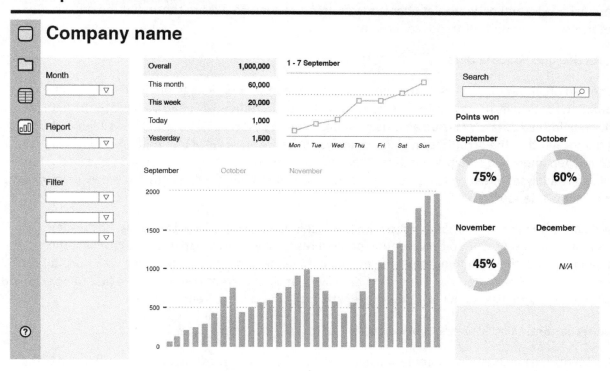

The laws around data are evolving. Privacy is a state of being that every organization must take responsibility for. Each organization must cloak its daily habits using a VPN (virtual private network) connection. A VPN service will scramble the signal so that identity and location are at least partially masked from trackers. A VPN will substantially reduce how much the world can observe the organization's online habits. Some of the most common reports used on a dashboard are new item trends, 52-week profit analysis, and exception reports. Dashboards can be customizable and present different views. Ideally, the data should all be from a single data

Identifying External Data Sources for Comparison

Benchmarking is another method that allows for the analysis of healthcare delivery, trends, and best practices. Benchmarks are useful in that they permit the comparison of apples to apples. This is especially true when audits are internal to an organization. Benchmarking allows the comparison of results with state, regional, or national organizations that are similar in structure. For example, the average length of stay or number of bed days may be a metric that is monitored and even tied to the performance of an organization.

Industry benchmarks in managed care organizations include: acute-care admissions per thousand; acute-care bed days per thousand; skilled nursing bed days per thousand; home care admissions per thousand; and home care visits per thousand. The benchmarking exercise can also help to identify processes that have an opportunity for improvement. The exercise supports monitoring of consistency in practice, while also enabling compliance with quality standards. Patients, caregivers, providers, payers, and a variety of other participants in the patient's care should be a part of evaluating their experience. Their feedback is critical in the evaluation of the overall effectiveness of a program.

The leadership team decides which benchmarks are appropriate for their organization and metrics. In most cases the benchmarks are standardized or mandated, as in Joint Commission benchmarks or national quality and patient safety benchmarks. Internal benchmarks are those that the organization determines are important trends to monitor.

Collecting and Validate Data

When an organization collects its own new data, despite best intentions to prevent data errors, somehow, data can still have mistakes. Therefore, the organization will need to validate the data by checking for bad data. Data from an outside source, such as the CDC, should still be validated once it is in the format that the organization plans to analyze it. There are a lot of unintentional mistakes that can occur when importing or exporting data. Therefore, it is important that data validation occurs before doing any analyses, creating tables, or reports from the data to be used, whether it is new data or data from an outside source.

Throughout the data validation process, the leadership team must always be asking the question, "Does this result make sense?" Typical validation procedures for continuous variables are checking the minimum value, the maximum value, the mean, and the median. Example: working with hospital data, one of the variables is a patient's length of time living at their current residence. The first thing is to find the minimum and maximum values for the length of time at their current address.

The results are: Min: .05 years Max: 47 years.

This seems reasonable; some people will have lived at their current address for a very long time, and others may have just moved into their home. If instead of getting those results, the following results were obtained: Min: 50 years Max 4.7 years there may have been some mathematical mistakes or data entered incorrectly.

When collecting and validating data, two main checks should be routinely done: double check that the data was downloaded properly, and check that the data was imported properly into the format for your analysis software. These are both steps where data mistakes can easily happen. Another useful data validation method is running cross tabulations (counting the number in each group of combinations of variables). This is useful because there are often combinations of variables that should not occur. Take, for example, the variables "sex" and "pregnancy status." One obvious combination that should never occur is a pregnant male. No matter how much effort is put into creating a good data collection system, errors will inevitably creep into the database making it necessary for data cleaning. Data cleaning can be intricate, time consuming, and costly, but it is a necessary step in any data-related project.

Measurement and Analysis

Using Data Management Systems

The amount of healthcare data available can be overwhelming. Healthcare leaders need to transition their operations to fit with a data-driven mentality. Administrators and physicians need to be diligent about collecting patient data, marketing departments need to shift towards basing their outreach on data, and patients need to be involved in their own care. Making data management a priority requires involvement from all players in the healthcare industry.

As the healthcare industry moves aggressively toward outcome-based reimbursement, all healthcare entities need to remodel their operations to focus on affordable, effective and accessible service delivery. Leaders are developing strategies to become more cost effective and more collaborative while meeting the security challenges of ever-evolving threats to their IT systems and data. It's important to find new ways to efficiently manage people, processes and technology to deliver integrated and effective care, as well as efficient business services.

The healthcare organization must also be able to adapt to new regulatory requirements and to rationalize and integrate systems in the wake of mergers and acquisitions or consolidation of payers and providers. Strategic thinking about the application of new technology can be important to controlling costs and optimizing IT value. Without a strategic approach, organizations run the risk of investing in solutions that neither integrate well with their enterprise nor optimize business value

Healthcare data management is the process of storing, protecting, and analyzing data pulled from diverse sources. Managing all of the available healthcare data allows health systems to create holistic views of patients, personalize treatments, improve communication, and enhance health outcomes. There are thousands of different data management systems and each organization must fit the Information Technology needs into both the fiscal plan and the operational plan each year. Senior leaders and IT management must work together to determine which products best meets the needs of the organization. A few of the data management systems include:

- Electronic Health Records (EHR): EHRs allow physicians and other medical personnel to record and store patient information electronically, simplifying the medical recording process for authorized users. With this tool, healthcare organizations are able to consolidate, centralize, and securely access patient medical data. The EHR replaces the paper medical charts and contains everything from physician orders and lab work to surgical notes and medications. Each patient has a specific record with unique identifiers.

- Healthcare Customer Relations Management (HCRM): A healthcare CRM has the ability to integrate, measure, analyze, and report on data from a variety of sources within one data hub. Specifically, this technology allows health systems to consolidate consumer and patient data from EHRs, engagement centers, social media, and many other sources. With CRM technology in place, healthcare organizations can develop a 360-degree view of patients that encompasses not only the patient lifecycle, but also includes consumer profiles, preferences, and behaviors.

- Reliability Centered Maintenance (RCM): A process that is generally used to achieve improvements in fields such as the establishment of safe minimum levels of maintenance. Successful implementation RCM leads to increase in cost effectiveness, reliability, machine uptime, and a greater understanding of the level of risk that the organization is managing. RCM can be used to create a cost-effective maintenance strategy that addresses the causes of equipment failure. The important functions of a piece of equipment with routine maintenance are identified, their dominant failure modes and causes determined, and the consequences of failure ascertained. Levels of criticality are assigned to the consequences of failure. Some functions are not critical and are left to "run to failure" while other functions must be preserved at all cost. This process directly addresses maintenance preventable failures. When the risk of such failures is very high, RCM encourages (and sometimes mandates) the user to consider changing something which will reduce the risk to a tolerable level. The result is a maintenance program that focuses scarce economic resources on those items that would cause the most trouble if they don't work.

- Enterprise application software (EAS): A computer software used to satisfy the needs of an organization rather than individual users. Such organizations include businesses, schools, interest-based user groups, clubs, charities, and governments. As enterprises have similar departments and systems in common, enterprise software is often available as a suite of customizable programs. Generally, the complexity of these tools requires specialist capabilities and specific knowledge. The software is intended to solve an enterprise-wide problem, rather than a departmental problem. EAS aims to improve the enterprise's productivity and efficiency by providing business logic support functionality. EAS is typically hosted on servers and provides simultaneous services to a large number of users, typically over a computer network. Services provided by enterprise software are typically business-oriented tools, such as:

  - Online and automated payment and billing processing
  - Security and Human Resources, Occupational Health and Safety
  - Project management
  - IT service management
  - Customer relationship management
  - Business intelligence

Using Tools to Display Data or Evaluate a Process

The most effective format for the dissemination and depiction of statistical data is often via a graph or chart. For those not familiar with data interpretation, visual tools such as Pareto charts, run charts, scattergrams, and control charts can easily depict the trends and correlational relationships between variables. Leadership teams will utilize appropriate tools to display data related to the organization's mission, values, and goals.

A Pareto chart depicts data in the form of bars placed in descending order, with a line representing the cumulative total. The 80-20 rule is a business rule of thumb that states that 80% of outcomes can be attributed to 20% of all causes for a given event. In business, the 80-20 rule is often used to point out that 80% of a company's revenue is generated by 20% of its total customers. Therefore, the rule is used to help managers identify and determine which operating factors are most important and should receive the most attention based on an efficient use of resources.

Supplementary quality control tools include the run chart, control charts, histograms, scatter plot diagrams, and check sheets. Both the run and the control charts are line graphs that depict data points along a continuum; however, the control chart includes a control limit. Both charts also clearly indicate trends and patterns of specific processes, and how well that process is performing. While control charts are best utilized when monitoring processes on an ongoing basis, run charts are best suited for investigating short-term process improvement activities.

Histograms graphically represent the variation of values within a group. This format depicts the center, spread, and shape of the data. The distribution will be distinctly normal, bi-modal, or skewed. One final format for depicting statistical data is the fishbone, or cause and effect diagram. Named or the shape, this diagram focuses largely on depicting the precipitating factors, or root causes, for a specific event or outcome. Those root causes can be separated into more meaningful categories. Practitioners can then engage in the brainstorming necessary to clarify potential solutions. This format for representing data is also useful when there is little quantitative data accessible for analysis.

Although every program and process evaluation project does not require the use of each tool, at least two charts are typically utilized for precision when reporting results. Each of these tools was described in more detail previously.

Using Statistics to Describe Data

Historically, statisticians utilize measures of central tendency when evaluating any set of data. The three most common measures of central tendency include the mean, median, and mode. The mean of the sample is the average of the sample, and is determined by adding all of the outcomes from the sample then dividing it by the total number of events. The median is the middle value within the data set when all results are presented in ascending or descending order. If the midpoint consists of two numbers, then the average is to be taken of the two. The mode is the most common value appearing within the data set. The range is the difference in the span of values within the complete set, or the largest value minus the smallest value. When a normal data set is generated, the data are depicted as a bell-shaped curve; the mean, median, and mode are the same.

Variance is the sum of the squared deviations from the mean, divided by the total size of the sample. The standard deviation is defined as the average distance of all points of data from the mean of the data set. The correlation, or dependent relationship between two quantitative continuous variables, can either be positive or negative. For example, if one variable increases corresponding to the increase of another, the two variables are said to be positively correlated. Alternatively, if one variable decreases while another increases, that relationship is considered to be negatively correlated. One additional measure, a t-test, is used to compare the differences between to the means of separate distributions. The t-test is a statistical tool that usually is done in Minitab or a similar software. It is generally thought to guide the determination of root causality between two processes.

Using Statistical Process Control

Statistical Process Control (SPC) is an industry-standard methodology for measuring and controlling quality during the manufacturing process. Quality data in the form of product or process measurements are obtained in real-time during manufacturing. This data is then plotted on a graph with pre-determined control limits. Control limits are determined by the capability of the process, whereas specification limits are determined by the client's needs. Data that falls within the control limits indicates that everything is operating as expected. Any variation within the control limits is likely due to a common cause—the natural variation that is expected as part of the process. If data falls outside of the control limits, this indicates that an assignable cause is likely the source of the product variation, and something within the process should be changed to fix the issue before defects occur. SPC dramatically reduces variability, improves productivity, reduces costs, and allows leaders to instantly react to process changes. Common areas of waste include scrap, rework, over-inspection, inefficient data collection, incapable machines and/or processes, paper-based quality systems and inefficient lines.

SPC has been a manufacturing standard for decades but it is only within the past 20 years that it has been used in healthcare. The thinking is that an error is an error and waste is waste, whether the process is patient related or material related. The process is what is important to control in order to reduce costs and eliminate rework.

Common cause variation, also called random variation, is the process by which numerous small general factors result in a specific effect on a process. These stressors to the process are predictable and occur in every process. For example, consider the effect of staffing in a typical emergency room. If it is determined that there is a thirty-minute wait for patients to be examined by a physician once admitted to an emergency room, the management can simply act to permanently increase staffing to the ER; or reduce the possibility of variance.

Special cause variation refers to the specific rare factors that can influence a process. These are new and unexpected stressors that occur sporadically. Considering the same example, special cause variation in this instance would be a wait of three hours for a patient to be examined once admitted to the ER. Upon further examination, the evaluator may uncover a specific event of staff being preoccupied caring for numerous patients involved in a local apartment building fire. The best way to solve this problem would be to institute disaster protocols, whereby specific individuals throughout the facility can be dispatched to the ER to manage the overflow when it does occur. Both interventions would require approaching the problem at its roots, engaging in corrective or preventative actions, and mitigating as much variation as possible.

A trend analysis is a method based on historical data about a process. There are no proven automatic techniques to identify in time series data; however, as long as the trend is consistently increasing or decreasing, the trend is evident. If the time series data contain considerable errors, then the first step in the process of trend identification is smoothing. Smoothing always involves some form of local averaging of data so that the nonsystematic components of individual observations cancel each other out. Medians can be used instead of means. The main advantage of median is that its results are less biased by outliers (within the smoothing window). Thus, if there are outliers in the data median smoothing typically produces smoother or more reliable curves.

Most time series patterns can be described in terms trend and seasonality. Trend represents a general systematic linear or nonlinear component that changes over time and does not repeat within the time range captured by the data. Seasonality may have a plateau followed by a period of exponential growth, however, it repeats itself in systematic intervals over time. For example, sales of a company can rapidly grow over years but they still follow consistent seasonal patterns.

Interpreting Data to Support Decision-Making

Once the leadership team has gathered, analyzed, and discussed the aggregated data they create a dialogue that will lead to the necessary changes. As the team interprets the data, they must keep in mind that a hypothesis cannot be proved true; one can only fail to reject the hypothesis. This means that no matter how much data the team collects, chance can always interfere with the results. Therefore, when interpreting the results of data, the leadership team must ask the following questions: Does the data answer our original question? How? Does the data help defend against any objections? How? Are there any limitation on our conclusions; any angles we haven't considered?

If the interpretation of the data holds up under all of these questions and considerations, then the team has come to a productive conclusion. The only remaining step is to use the results of the data analysis process to decide a best course of action. With practice, data analysis gets faster and more accurate – meaning better, more-informed decisions can be made to run the organization most effectively.

Comparing Data Sources to Establish Benchmarks

The cornerstone of data management is to ensure that the organization is reaching pre-determined goals. Benchmarking in healthcare is defined as the continual and collaborative discipline of measuring and comparing the results of key work processes. Typically, the ideas and practices of the best performers are compared with the host organization. The four distinct types of benchmarking for quality improvement include:

- Internal: comparing equivalent processes within the same organization
- Competitive: comparing similar processes to a competitor within the same industry
- Functional: comparing similar processes to those in different industries
- Generic: comparing the general concepts of processes in unrelated industries

Staff progress can be measured internally and the separate business functions can be compared externally. Leadership within the organization can employ comparative analysis on a cyclical, weekly, or daily basis in an effort to respond to concerns in real-time, rather than after the impact has reached the consumer.

It will be necessary to have frequent brainstorming sessions. Brainstorming can be referred to as a way of using a selected group of individuals to rapidly produce, clarify, and evaluate ideas or problems. Staff must be encouraged to preview the preliminary data and leadership must allow for an open-ended and honest critique of what does and does not work. It is important to note that the purpose of any brainstorming session is to generate as many ideas as possible. There are no right or wrong answers, as the object is to generate momentum around finding solutions. Brainstorming offers the team an opportunity to view all aspects of the problem and can often yield unexpected results. Results shared within the organization help each employee to connect with the results and recognize that they can affect change through their individual behaviors.

Internal benchmarking efforts encourage top performers to form more practical solutions to problems articulated by the data. Competitive benchmarking can help delineate how similar organizations solved similar defects. The comparative analysis can also reveal how the current processes are outpacing the competitors, which encourages the integration of what works with what does not work well enough. This approach will help the leadership team to deliver on the promise of providing exceptional care.

Participating in External Reporting

Once the leadership team has established the overall mission and goals of the healthcare organization, the next step will be to ensure that quality and safety activities are in alignment with those goals. Data gleaned from the internal and competitive benchmarking and brainstorming sessions are meant to transform processes and procedures that have no statistically significant value added to the business. Aggregated data must be analyzed to reveal trends in the data that indicate which of the organizations' established goals and objectives can be translated into critical success factors. These are then used to create KPI—measurable data that will further indicate if the goals and objectives are attainable. The data or input measures are typically representative of services or skill level, whereas output measures represent outcomes and results.

The Healthcare Effectiveness Data and Information Set (HEDIS) is a group of performance standards that the majority of health plans adhere to in an effort to standardize the overall vision quality of care delivered to patients. These standards include areas related to quality of care, access to care, and member satisfaction. In its entirety, HEDIS comprises a total of 94 diverse measures across seven specific types of care. This data information set allows for equanimity among organizations and health plans and creates a more competitive approach to meeting the numerous quality standards among healthcare systems. Health plans can utilize the reported results to gauge their performance against those reported by competitors. This comparison tool is a registered and trademarked strategy of the National Committee for Quality Assurance (NCQA). This data clearinghouse allows for an internal benchmark, as health plans can review their own previous results and identify upward and downward trends. The Quality Compass is an interactive web-based tool within the NCQA arsenal that generates quality reports based on specific plans, benchmarks, and time frames.

One additional facet of the HEDIS quality standards is the Consumer Assessment of Healthcare Providers and Systems (CAHPS) survey, which was developed in 1995 as a method for quantifying members' satisfaction regarding their overall experience with specific health plans. The general public had previously struggled to locate information regarding the standards of quality achieved and the members' subsequent satisfaction. The NCQA encourages the exchange of quality information to consumers who can view both quality adherence statistics and accreditation standards. By viewing the State of Health Care Quality report, consumers are better equipped to monitor the report cards of healthcare plans and organizations. Completed annually, the primary goal of this quality report is focused improvement of the dissemination, implementation, and spread of evidence-based care across the country.

CMS, commercial health plans, and private physicians, as well as healthcare leaders and legislators, worked diligently to develop the Core Quality Measure Collaborative. The core quality measures were developed to promote evidence-based care, decrease healthcare expenditures, and encourage providers to utilize bundling of services.

Bundled payments, also known as episode of care payment or package pricing, can be defined as a single payment made to cover the costs of the treatment provided for any given service. Led by the America's Health Insurance Plans (AHIP), this initiative was established to encourage payers to employ a set of core measures to utilize during reporting. The Core Measures include the following: Cardiology, Gastroenterology, HIV and Hepatitis C, Medical Oncology, Obstetrics and Gynecology, Orthopedics, Pediatrics, Accountable Care Organizations, Patient Centered Medical Homes, and Primary Care. It is important to note that the primary purpose of reporting significant findings is the adherence to specific standards of excellence.

Practice Questions

1. Which statement BEST describes the Lean Six Sigma approach to process improvement?
    a. The Lean Six Sigma approach can be defined as the continual and collaborative discipline of measuring and comparing the results of key work processes
    b. A plan to eliminate or lower the likelihood of an error, or to make the occurrence of an error so obvious that any possibility of that error impacting the consumer is practically impossible
    c. The primary goal is to produce more effective processes, policies, and procedures that reduce variation and significantly lower the chances of negative outcomes
    d. A specific methodology that calculates the true costs of a potential solution compared to the actual benefits

2. Which statement BEST describes the purpose of the project charter?
    a. The primary goal is to determine the ability of a specific process to deliver value as required by the customer
    b. This written agreement usually includes: primary reason for the project; the goal and scope of the project; the expected budget and roles of each member of the team
    c. The written agreement that acts as measurable data to indicate if the goals and objectives of the project are attainable
    d. The primary goal is to produce more effective processes, policies, and procedures that reduce variation and significantly lower the chances of negative outcomes

3. Which is the BEST description for the acronym SIPOC?
    a. Supplier, inputs, process, outputs, customer
    b. Supporter, inputs, process, outcomes, consumer
    c. Supplier, improvement, product, outputs, consumer
    d. Supporters, inputs, products, outcomes, consumer

4. What is the major difference between scorecards and dashboards?
    a. Scorecards involve comparing equivalent processes within the same organization; dashboards can be comparing similar processes to a competitor within the same industry
    b. Scorecards are a single payment made to cover the costs of the treatment provided for any given treatment; dashboards are written agreements that act as measurable data to indicate if the goals and objectives of the project are attainable
    c. Scorecards can be defined as a written account that compares and measures the performance of specific individuals against the projected goals of the organization; dashboards are quality measurement tools that actually allow the management team to visually analyze the KPI of each specific individual within the healthcare team
    d. Scorecards can be defined as the passive and unplanned spread of new practices; dashboards are defined as the active spread of those new practices to a target audience utilizing planned methodologies

5. Which of the following is true regarding data management?
    a. It is only done by IT personnel
    b. It is always done on local servers
    c. It is done via cloud based systems
    d. It involves acquiring, validating, storing, protecting, and processing data

6. In order to secure electronic files and reports, the clinician must do which of the following?
   a. Use computer screen locks and shortened time-out locks
   b. Use black-out screens whenever the computer is left unattended
   c. Limit access to computers
   d. All of the above

7. The IHI Simple Data Collection Plan begins data collection planning by first doing which of the following?
   a. Asking why these data are being collected
   b. Deciding the tools to use
   c. Deciding on team members
   d. Setting goals

8. What do process measures show?
   a. If the team met their goals
   b. How the steps in the system perform
   c. If the measures improved care
   d. All of the above

9. What do control charts tell the team?
   a. The control limit of the process
   b. What processes are out of control
   c. If they met their goals
   d. How a process changes over time

10. What does a trend analysis help the team do best?
    a. Decide which trend to follow
    b. Understand historical data about a process.
    c. Identify the mean, median, and mode
    d. Prove a hypothesis

11. What is the BEST description of a correlation?
    a. A correlation is a dependent relationship between two quantitative continuous variables and can either be positive or negative
    b. A correlation is a way of using a selected group of individuals to rapidly produce, clarify, and evaluate ideas or problems
    c. A correlation is an independent relationship between two quantitative continuous variables and can either be positive or negative
    d. A correlation is defined as the continual and collaborative discipline of measuring and comparing the results of key work processes

12. Which quality control tool is best suited to use when investigating short-term process improvement activities?
    a. Run charts
    b. T-tests
    c. Control charts
    d. Pareto charts

13. What does the acronym DMAIC refer to in the Lean Six Sigma project management model?
    a. Describe, manage, accountability, interpret, and compare
    b. Define, manage, analyze, interpret, and control
    c. Describe, measure, analyze, improve, and compare
    d. Define, measure, analyze, improve, and control

14. According to the Lean Six Sigma framework, which two quality tools are typically utilized in the analyze phase?
    a. Run charts and Pareto charts
    b. Process capability assessments and critical to quality trees
    c. Project charter and process mapping
    d. Brainstorming and benchmarking

15. What is the best description of positive correlation depicted in a scattergram?
    a. If one variable decreases while another increases, that relationship is considered to be a negative correlation; the points on the scatter plot will be close together and trend to the left in the form of a line
    b. No correlation would yield a value of zero, with the data on the scatter plot appearing to have no actual clear shape or direction within the middle of the axes
    c. If one variable increases while another increases, that relationship is considered to be a positive correlation; the points on the scatter plot will be close together and trend to the right in the form of a line
    d. If one variable increases while another increases up to a certain point, that relationship is considered to be a curvilinear correlation; the data points will resemble a checkmark

16. What is the purpose of the Healthcare Effectiveness Data and Information Set (HEDIS)?
    a. A correlation is defined as the continual and collaborative discipline of measuring and comparing the results of key work processes
    b. A group of performance standards that the majority of health plans adhered to in an effort to standardize the overall vision quality of care delivered to patients
    c. The written agreement that acts as measurable data to indicate if the goals and objectives of the project are attainable
    d. The primary goal is to produce more effective processes, policies, and procedures that reduce variation and significantly lower the chances of negative outcomes

17. What is the best description of statistical process control?
    a. The continual and collaborative discipline of measuring and comparing the results of key work processes
    b. The process by which numerous small general factors result in a specific effect on a process
    c. The specific rare factors that can influence a process
    d. A strategy for instituting ongoing process improvement

18. What is the BEST description of a critical to quality tree?
    a. This quality control tool helps to emphasize the frequency of the most impactful problems in order to allocate the appropriate amount of resources to rectify the problem
    b. Critical to quality trees graphically represent the variation of values within a group; this format depicts the center, spread, and shape of the data
    c. Critical to quality trees can be defined as the specific measurable facets of a process whose performance standards must be met to satisfy the customer
    d. This tool helps the CPHQ professional to determine the purpose, roles, scope, and budget of the investigation

19. What is the best method of noting quantitative or qualitative data?
    A. Scorecards
    b. Check sheets
    c. Fishbone diagrams
    d. KPI

20. Which statistical quality tool would be the BEST choice to depict the center, spread, and shape of data?
    a. Histograms
    b. Run chart
    c. Control charts
    d. Fishbone diagram

21. What is the difference between common cause variation and special cause variation?
    a. Common cause variation is the process by which numerous small general factors result in a specific effect on a process; special cause variation refers to the specific rare factors that can influence a process
    b. Common cause variation is the process of comparing equivalent processes within the same organization; special cause variation refers to comparing similar processes to a competitor within the same industry
    c. Common cause variation can be defined as the passive and unplanned spread of new practices; special cause variation is defined as the active spread of those new practices to target audience utilizing planned methodologies
    d. Common cause variation is the process by which a single payment is made to cover the costs of the treatment provided for any given treatment; special cause variation refers to measurable data that will further indicate if the goals and objectives are attainable

22. Outcome measures tell the organization how the system impacts which of the following?
    a. The organizational goals and values
    b. HEDIS measures
    c. Accreditation measures
    d. Values of patients and others

23. What is the industry-standard methodology for measuring and controlling quality during the manufacturing process in real-time with pre-determined control limits called?
    a. Lean manufacturing
    b. Statistical Process Control (SPC)
    c. Variability Index
    d. Quality Control (QC)

24. What are two steps where data mistakes happen most often?
    a. Entering and collating
    b. Saving and editing
    c. Downloading and importing
    d. All of the above

25. Non-probability Sampling is:
    a. based on human choice
    b. volunteer samples
    c. sources of bias
    d. All of the above

26. What is the term for tendency of a statistic to overestimate or underestimate a parameter?
    a. Central tendency
    b. Bias
    c. Smoothing
    d. Common cause variation

27. Which of the following is/are true regarding Informed Consent forms?
    a. They must be completed at admission
    b. They must be signed, dated, and witnessed
    c. They must be maintained under lock and key
    d. All of the above are true

28. What are the four types of benchmarking?
    a. Investigative, internal, external, and generic
    b. Internal, cooperative, external, and competitive
    c. Internal, competitive, functional, and generic
    d. Intensive, competitive, functional, and generic

29. What is the BEST description of brainstorming?
    a. Brainstorming is defined as the continual and collaborative discipline of measuring and comparing the results of key work processes
    b. Brainstorming can be referred to as a written account that compares and measures the performance of specific individuals against the projected goals of the organization
    c. Brainstorming can best be defined as the rate at which newly disseminated ideas or innovations are adopted and implemented
    d. Brainstorming can be referred to as a way of using a selected group of individuals to rapidly produce, clarify, and evaluate ideas or problems

30. Which statement BEST describes the purpose of bundled payments?
    a. This initiative was established to encourage payers to employ a set of core measures to utilize during reporting
    b. The primary goal is to produce more effective processes, policies, and procedures that reduce variation and significantly lower the chances of negative outcomes
    c. This initiative depicts the active spread of those new practices to a target audience, utilizing planned methodologies
    d. This initiative can best be defined as measurable data that will further indicate if the goals and objectives of the project are attainable

Answers Explanations

1. C: The primary goal of Lean Six Sigma is to produce more effective processes, policies, and procedures that reduce variation and significantly lower the chances of negative outcomes.

2. B: The project charter is a written agreement that usually includes that primary reason for the project, the goal and scope of the project, and the expected budget and roles of each member of the team.

3. A: Choice *A* is correct; it is the meaning of the acronym.

4. C: Scorecards can be defined as a written account that compares and measures the performance of specific individuals against the projected goals of the organization; dashboards are quality measurement tools that actually allow the management team to visually analyze the KPI of each specific individual within the healthcare team.

5. D: Data management involves acquiring, validating, storing, protecting, and processing data.

6. D: In order to secure electronic files and reports, the clinician must use computer screen locks and shortened time-out locks, use black-out screens whenever the computer is left unattended, and limit access to computers.

7. A: The IHI Simple Data Collection Plan begins data collection planning by first asking why data are being collected. Additional questions to consider include things like what type of data will be necessary, what data analysis tools will be used to display that obtained data, and where/how can the data be obtained?

8. B: Process measures show the steps in the system perform.

9. D: Control charts show a process changes over time. As line graphs, they clearly indicate trends and patterns of specific processes, and how well that process is performing.

10. B: A trend analysis helps the team understand historical data about a process.

11. A: A correlation is a dependent relationship between two quantitative continuous variables and can either be positive or negative.

12. A: Run charts are best suited to investigate short-term process improvement activities. Like control charts, they are line graphs that indicate trends and patterns of specific processes, and how well that process is performing.

13. D: DMAIC stands for define, measure, analyze, improve, and control. The DMAIC model helps improve existing processes and allows for the methodical development of an action plan to streamline and standardize laborious processes, reduce waste, and mitigate risks to the patient population in any healthcare setting.

14. A: The run and Pareto charts are most frequently used in the analyze stage.

15. C: A positive correlation occurs when one variable increases while another increases; the points on the scatterplot will be close together and trend to the right in the form of a line.

16. B: The HEDIS is a group of performance standards that the majority of health plans adhere to in an effort to standardize the overall vision quality of care delivered to patients.

17. D: Statistical process control is a strategy for instituting ongoing process improvement. It is the industry-standard methodology for measuring and controlling quality during the manufacturing process in real-time with pre-determined control limits.

18. C: Critical to quality trees can be defined as the specific measurable facets of a process whose performance standards must be met to satisfy the customer.

19. B: Check sheets are best for notating data for collection when data can be collected by the same person at the same time.

20. A: Histograms are the best format to depict the center, spread, and shape of aggregated data.

21. A: Common cause variation is the process by which numerous small general factors result in a specific effect on a process; special cause variation refers to the specific rare factors that can influence a process.

22. D: Outcome measures tell the organization how the system impacts the values of patients and others. They reflect the impact of the health care service or intervention on the health status of patients served. While they may seem to represent the gold standard in measuring quality, an outcome is the result of numerous factors, many beyond providers' control.

23. B: Statistical Process Control is the industry-standard methodology for measuring and controlling quality during the manufacturing process in real-time with pre-determined control limits.

24. C: Downloading and importing are the two areas where most data mistakes occur.

25. D: Non-probability sampling should be avoided because it involves volunteer samples and haphazard (convenience) samples, which are based on human choice rather than random selection. Statistical theory cannot explain how the samples might behave and potential sources of bias are rampant.

26. B: Bias is the tendency of a statistic to overestimate or underestimate a parameter. It can occur from sampling or measurement errors, or by using unrepresentative samples. If the statistic is unbiased, the average of all statistics from all samples will average the true population parameter.

27. D: Informed consent form must be completed at admission. They must be signed, dated, and witnessed, and maintained under lock and key.

28. C: The four types of benchmarking are internal, competitive, functional, and generic.

29. D: Brainstorming can be referred to as a way of using a selected group of individuals to rapidly produce, clarify, and evaluate ideas or problems.

30. A: Bundled payments were established to encourage payers to employ a set of core measures to utilize during reporting.

Performance and Process Improvement

Identifying Opportunities for Improvement

Facilitating Discussion About Quality Improvement Opportunities

A facilitator plans, guides, and manages a group event to ensure that the objectives are met effectively, with clear thinking, good participation and full buy-in from everyone involved. An effective facilitator must be objective, meaning that for the purposes of the group process, the facilitator takes a neutral stance. Focus must be purely on the group process.

Group process is the approach used to manage discussions, obtain input from all team members, and bring the event through to a successful conclusion. Great facilitation occurs when the group process produces ideas, solutions, and decisions. In order to accomplish these goals, the facilitator must design and plan the group process and select the tools that will help the group progress towards that outcome. The facilitator will guide and control the group process to ensure that: there is effective participation; participants achieve a consensus; all contributions are considered and included in the ideas, solutions or decisions that emerge; members take shared responsibility for the outcome; and that outcomes, actions and questions are properly recorded and actioned, and appropriately dealt with afterwards.

Some items a facilitator needs to consider:

- Do you want an open discussion, or a structured process?
- Can you cover the variety of topics needed?
- Can you generate enough ideas and solutions?
- And can you involve everyone, and get their buy-in?
- The number of participants.
- The nature of the topics under discussion.
- The type of involvement people need to have.
- The background and positions of the participants.
- How well they know the subject and each other.
- The time available.

The following are some of the tools and techniques that can help the facilitator run an effective meeting or event:

- Ice Breakers – Easing group contribution.
- MultiVoting – Choosing fairly between many options.
- Brainstorming – Generating many radical ideas.
- Role Playing – Preparing for difficult situations.
- Small group discussion
- Paired listening
- Parking space
- Urgent/non-urgent grid
- Pros and cons list
- Plus-Minus-Implications list

The final stage of preparation is to think about how the meeting will be controlled and divided.

The facilitator should set the ground rules: What rules should participants follow? How will he or she ensure that people respect each other's ideas? How will questions be handled? The facilitator should prepare some ground rules in advance, and propose and seek agreement to these at the start of the event. The facilitator should do the following?

- Set the scene. Run through the objectives and agenda. Make sure that everyone understands their role, and what the group is seeking to achieve.

- Get things flowing. Make sure that everyone introduces themselves, or use appropriate icebreakers to get the meeting off to a positive start.

- Keep up the momentum and energy. Intervene as the proceedings and energy levels proceed. Make sure that people remain focused and interested.

- Listen, engage, and include. Stay alert, listen actively, and remain interested and engaged. This sets a good example for other participants, and also means you are always ready to intervene in facilitative ways.

- Monitor checkpoints, and summarize. Keep in control of the agenda, tell people what they've achieved and what's next. Summarize often. Intervene only if absolutely required.

- Remind the group what has been discussed, and keep them focused and moving forward. When in doubt, ask for clarification before the discussion moves on.

- After the event, follow up to ensure that outstanding actions and issues are progressed, and that the proceedings are brought to a successful conclusion.

- Last but not least, among the responsibilities of a facilitator is the recording of outputs, and of bringing these together, sharing them, and making sure they are actioned.

Before sending out a meeting invite, it is important to define the objective that the meeting is going to achieve. Clearly and precisely stating the objective in advance helps determine who should attend, the likely duration, the agenda items. This is also a useful opportunity to consider whether a meeting is the most appropriate technique, or if other techniques such as interviews, observation, workshop, or scenario analysis would be preferable.

The facilitator must define and articulate the objectives (discuss improvement opportunities for next year) but also the tangible outcomes or outputs that the team aims to achieve. This sets expectations and will ensure that people know precisely what is expected. If these outcomes are achieved, then the meeting is a success. If not, it may be necessary to reconvene or reconsider a different approach.

A good agenda may only have a few action items. It is better to focus on broad objectives first and drill down to more specific objectives. As an example:

1. Brainstorm session: What worked well this year and what didn't? (15 min)
2. Determine priority items down to top five (10 min)
3. Action plans for the top 3 (20 min)
4. Questions/concerns/next steps (10 min)

When working in a complex stakeholder landscape, there is a temptation to invite everyone to the meeting. The facilitator must be selective because large groups can become very hard to manage. Our stakeholders' time is precious so we should use it effectively. The facilitator should limit the group to a number between 5 and 20 people. Persons who have expressed an interest in the topic, people with power, people with knowledge of the task at hand, are all good choices for team members.

Preparation for meetings is essential. The facilitator should have a clear and concise agenda, get the information out well in advance of the meeting, and it may be necessary to personally brief attendees. If there is a possibility of conflict, the facilitator must understanding why in advance and have a plan to deescalate any conflict.

The facilitator must assign a scribe who can also help with any logistical items. Ensure that the meeting room is booked and large enough, equipment (projector, flip-charts, slides) is available and working, and that the facilitator has notes and anything else needed for the meeting.

Running a successful meeting is only useful if the outcomes and actions have follow-up. Ensuring there are clear actions, process owners, and review dates will the team succeed. Simple action steps, when well-managed, go a long way to ensuring that items receive appropriate follow-up.

When a decision is made to initiate a performance or process improvement project, healthcare organizations typically begin by reviewing all areas of weakness. Primarily, those areas are determined by reviewing the business goals, mission, vision, and values of the organization, along with the associated key performance indicators (KPIs). The basic framework of the project is built on this needs assessment. It is also necessary to determine the critical to quality measures (CTQs), which are the aspects of a business process or product that must be met in order to satisfy the consumer. Once a significant list has been compiled, the team can then begin to clearly define the problem.

Ideally, organizations seeking to maintain a high level of excellence should consider evaluating the internal voice of the business (VOB). The VOB can be regarded as the implicit and explicit needs and requirements of the business, such as profit, competitive edge, and growth. When designing an appropriate process flow for a client-centered service, it will be crucial to determine the must have aspects of that service according to the customer, or the voice of the customer (VOC). The consumer's voice is the outward image of the business, and the reputation that the business has earned among consumers. Building on the external VOC and the internal VOB, the project management team must work collaboratively to ensure that performance and production waste are eliminated, while simultaneously improving overall organizational efficiency and revenue. When standards and policies that were originally created to satisfy the customer according to the CTQs are not consistently met, the business begins to falter. It is important to ascertain whether the projected business goals meet or exceed the VOC and VOB, or whether they have competing or conflicting interests.

When the business's needs do not match the customer's needs, resources can become exhausted. The team will conduct a needs assessment based on the priority of CTQs to calculate how projected goals from previous quarters differ from current results. These needs assessments are performed throughout the company and on all crucial processes and procedures. Specialized departments that handle more intricate issues may have a more stringent process and procedure assessment schedule. Apparent gaps in outcomes related to the VOC and the VOB must be addressed and the staff retrained in an effort to standardize policies, procedures, and processes. Addressing CTQs enables the project management team to focus on the problem.

Assisting with Establishing Priorities

It is impractical and unnecessary to monitor all care all the time, so priority should be given to those aspects of care that are high volume, high risk, and problem prone. Priority setting should reflect the mix of services and problems of each organization. Judgments concerning quality must be as objective as possible and must grow out of a combined process of screening and peer review. The leadership team must pay particular attention to gaining a common understanding of the definition of high quality care, utilizing review programs that are continuous, priority-oriented, and effective. The 80/20 rule must also be acknowledged and investigated. All indicators and criteria used to monitor care must be consistent with current state-of-the-art practice. Leaders must invest time and funds to improving diffusion of current clinical knowledge to practitioners. They must be equally aware that substandard care may occur and seek new ways to improve that care.

The efforts to control costs of health care are well chronicled, and they range from exclusion of services from reimbursement to cost sharing, prospective pricing, managed care, and expansion in the options of health plans from which employers and employees can choose. The broad scope of these efforts to control health care costs and the vigor with which they are pursued are now prompting questions about the resulting impact on quality. Also, faced with the need to make choices between a number of health care plans, employers and employees want to know the differences in quality between the competitors, and they are beginning to clarify the parameters of health care that are most important to them.

It is recognized that a substantial and expanding proportion of care is provided outside the inpatient units of hospitals and that the care in such settings greatly impacts on the ability of the hospital to provide high quality inpatient care and vice versa. The most effective way to review and improve the quality of care is to track patients through an episode of illness rather than to concentrate attention on just one setting in a continuum of care.

To succeed, quality evaluation must be an integral component of the operation of any health care organization and must receive the consistent attention and support of the leaders of governing body, management, and clinical staff. The full scope of the organization's clinical services must be analyzed for possible inclusion in the monitoring activity. Indicators of high or low quality must be identified for each aspect of care. Thresholds for evaluation can then be established for each indicator. The table below shows a few examples of indicators for important aspects of care, by type of care:

Ambulatory care	Inpatient care	Home care	Long-term care /Hospice care
Alcoholism treatment	Discharge planning	Medication reconciliation	Effective control of the symptoms of cancer
Adequate prenatal care, intra- and postpartum care	Pain Control	Continuity of care	Nutritional needs
Adequate foot care in diabetic	Communication	Fall prevention	Pain control

Even in the best of organizations, unwanted and unwarranted events occur. Reducing their incidence will require a combination of patience and pressure; the challenge is to gauge when to apply each. The philosophy that will usually be most effective in improving quality will be to expect diligent, professionally sound, continuous monitoring of quality and rapid identification and correction of problems where they are found. Understanding that perfection in health care is impossible to achieve, our constant goal should be to do better today than we did yesterday. Pareto analysis can show how the 10 most costly care process families account for 48 percent of the direct variable cost in that health system. By identifying the most costly areas of care and studying the variations, you now have potential areas to focus on. Variation in direct variable cost is a good surrogate for variation in quality of care. Valuable information like this gives health systems a starting point. Follow the data and focus on the top clinical families. Once those care processes have improved, move on to others. Once there is consensus on priorities, the clinical teams can help determine the best ways to reduce variation while improving care at the same time.

Facilitating Development of Action Plans or Projects

Identifying activities doesn't make the action plan, which needs to be more than the enumeration of activities that will be carried out. An action plan should include: a time frame; an evaluation of the existing capacities to be used to identify missing capacities ; a cost evaluation; identification of the actors; appropriate mechanisms for monitoring and assessing progress. In other words, five W's and H – who what, when where, why, and how.

The purpose (outcome) for each objective has to be identified as well as the outputs. The Action Plan should be inserted in a logical framework reflecting the intervention logic of the strategy for the development of statistics. The framework for the action plan might include:

- Overall objective: the broad development impact to which the project contributes

- Outcome: the development outcome at the end of the NSDS implementation; more specifically, the expected benefits to the target groups

- Outputs: the direct and tangible results (goods and services) that will be delivered, which are largely under the project management control

- Activities: the tasks that need to be carried out to deliver the planned results and expected dates of completion

- Indicators: linked to the objective-based planning and measure how the objectives, purpose, results, and activities will be achieved

An action plan should be detailed and used as a daily instrument for the team leader. It should be used to control the actions, costs and timeline, to monitor and evaluate the implementation, to make necessary adjustments and to assess the results. The work program should be underpinned by a budget, to control operations and results. The budget is crucial for the implementation of the action plans. All the actions need to be carefully budgeted to have an overview of the total cost of the action plan and to identify the ways to contain cost.

Example of an Action Plan

Goal 1	Action Step Descriptions	Party/Dept Responsible	Date to begin	Date due
Write your goal statement here				
List resources and desired outcomes				

Goal 2	Action Step Descriptions	Party/Dept Responsible	Date to begin	Date due
Write your goal statement here				
List resources and desired outcomes				

Goal 3	Action Step Descriptions	Party/Dept Responsible	Date to begin	Date due
Write your goal statement here				
List resources and desired outcomes				

Goal 4	Action Step Descriptions	Party/Dept Responsible	Date to begin	Date due
Write your goal statement here				
List resources and desired outcomes				

Facilitating Implementation of Performance Improvement Methods

As mentioned earlier, there are four terms that apply to starting a new process or method in an organization:

1. *Diffusion* is the passive and unplanned spread of new practices.

2. *Dissemination* is the active spread of new practices to a target audience utilizing planned methodologies.

3. *Implementation* occurs when those practices are adopted and integrated within a healthcare setting.

4. *Spread* refers to the rate at which newly disseminated ideas or innovations are adopted and implemented.

Although QI models vary in approach and methods, a basic underlying principle is that QI is a continuous activity, not a one-time thing. As change is implemented there will always be issues to address and challenges to manage; things are never perfect. Lessons learned can be used to shift strategy and try new interventions.

Plan-Do-Study-Act Model

Plan Strategy

Prepare for change : create team and establish/confirm goals

Investigate potential interventions

Reassess & Respond

Use CAHPS data to asses what worked, what didn't

Spread successful innovations

Develop, Test Strategy

Select measures to monitor progress

Develop changes

Conduct small tests to change

Adapt changes to organizational context

Identity and deal with barriers

Monitor Strategy

Implement changes and hold the gains

Evaluate progress against criteria

<u>PDSA</u>

The fundamental approach that serves as the basis for most process improvement models in healthcare is the PDSA cycle, which stands for Plan, Do, Study, Act. As illustrated in in the figure above, this cycle is a systematic series of steps for learning and continual improvement of a product or process. Underlying the concept of PDSA is the idea that systems are made up of interdependent, interacting elements that are unpredictable and nonlinear in operation. Therefore, small changes can have large effects on the system. The PDSA cycle involves all staff in assessing problems and suggesting and testing potential solutions. This bottom-up approach increases the likelihood that staff will embrace the changes, a key requirement for successful QI.

The PDSA model has four parts.

1. **Plan.** This step involves identifying a goal or purpose, formulating an intervention or theory for change, defining success metrics, and putting a plan into action. When using PDSA to improve a process, the first step is to Identify possible goals and strategies to implement. A goal should reflect the specific aspects of performance that the team is targeting. It should also be measurable and feasible. By setting this goal, the team will be able to clearly communicate objectives to all of the sectors in your organization that you might need to support or help implement the intervention.

With objectives in place, the next task is to identify possible interventions and select one that seems promising. To decide which new ideas or benchmark practices to implement, the improvement team needs to consider several factors such as compatibility with the organization and local culture. The ideas must have technical merit because those that are most likely to be adopted are those that provide significant advantages over existing practices for patients and providers. The best intervention will be one that fits with the problem. It must suit the specific problem to be addressed. To ensure a good fit, the improvement team should seek input from both affected staff as well as patients or members. If either source of information is ignored during planning, the chosen intervention may not fix the real problem.

The team can produce visual displays of the team performance over time by tracking the metric on control or run charts. Control and run charts are helpful tools for regularly assessing the impact of process improvement and redesign efforts: monthly, weekly, or even daily. In contrast to tables of aggregated data which present an overall picture of performance at a given point in time, run and control charts offer an ongoing record of the impact of process changes over time. Dashboard reports are another way to display performance.

2. **Do.** This is the step in which the components of the plan are implemented. Prepare a written action plan for your organization. State the goals, list the strategies to achieve those goals, and then delineate the specific actions needed to implement the selected interventions to address the identified problems. It also helps to lay out the calendar for all actions in a Gantt chart format, so the timing of actions makes sense and is feasible to complete. Seek a feasible number of measures that address the most important aspects of the improvements you are trying to achieve. Too many measures could create a burden on the staff, leading to loss of attention due to information overload; too few measures may omit tracking of important aspects of the changes you are making.

3. **Study.** This step involves monitoring outcomes to test the validity of the plan for signs of progress and success, or problems and areas for improvement. Short-cycle, small-scale tests, coupled with analysis of test results, are helpful because microsystems or teams can learn from these tests before they implement actions more broadly. Small-scale tests of the interventions you wish to implement help

refine improvements by incorporating small modifications over time. Conducting these small tests of change can be very powerful. They allow for incremental modifications of interventions to fix problems, which helps the larger implementation run smoothly. Failures are low-risk because you have not tried to change the entire culture. Enthusiasm and positive word-of-mouth acknowledge early successes. It is easier to accumulate evidence for implementation when people are engaged in making something work rather than focused on the failure analysis. Most improvement strategies require some adaptation to the culture of the organization. Patient-centered improvement strategies have to consider the needs of patients and their families as well as the staff. Moreover, front-line staff will frequently resist new ideas if they are not allowed to modify them and test their own ideas.

4. **Act.** This step closes the cycle, integrating the learning generated by the entire process, which can be used to adjust the goal, change methods, or even reformulate an intervention or improvement initiative altogether. Implementation is expanded to reach sustainable improvement. Building off of the development and testing of specific changes, the final stage of the PDSA cycle involves adopting the intervention and evaluating it against the goals of the improvement project and the measures established for tracking improvement progress. This part of the improvement cycle is the ongoing work of health care and where teams spend most of their time. There are no set rules about how long this part of the cycle takes. Most monitoring takes place on a monthly or quarterly basis.

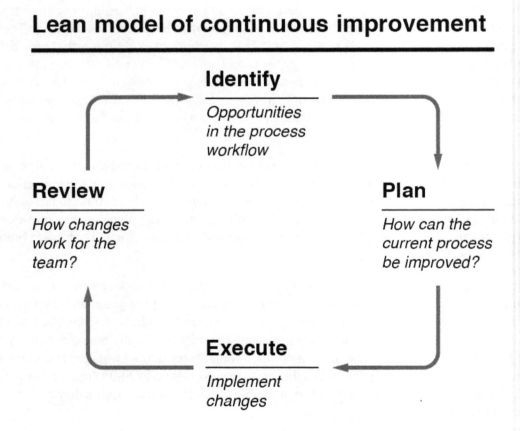

Lean model of continuous improvement

Identify

Opportunities in the process workflow

Review

How changes work for the team?

Plan

How can the current process be improved?

Execute

Implement changes

<u>Six Sigma and Lean</u>

Lean Six Sigma is a fact-based, data-driven philosophy of improvement that values defect prevention over defect detection. It drives customer satisfaction and bottom-line results by reducing variation, waste, and cycle time. It also promotes the use of work standardization and flow, thereby creating a competitive advantage. It applies anywhere variation and waste exist, and every employee should be involved. The Six Sigma perspective views all work as processes that can be defined, measured, analyzed, improved and controlled. Processes require inputs (x) and they produce outputs (y). If the inputs are controlled, the outputs will be controlled. This is generally expressed as $y = f(x)$.

The demarcation between Six Sigma and Lean has blurred. We are hearing about terms such as "Lean Six Sigma" with greater frequency because process improvement requires aspects of both approaches to attain positive results. Six Sigma focuses on reducing process variation and enhancing process control, whereas lean drives out waste (non-value-added) and promotes work standardization and flow. Lean and Six Sigma have the same general purpose of providing the customer with the best possible quality, cost, delivery, and a newer attribute, nimbleness. The two initiatives approach their common purpose from slightly different angles: Lean focuses on waste reduction, whereas Six Sigma emphasizes variation reduction. Lean achieves its goals by using less technical tools such as kaizen, workplace organization, and visual controls, whereas Six Sigma tends to use statistical data analysis, design of experiments, and hypothesis tests.

The most successful users have begun with the Lean approach, making the workplace as efficient and effective as possible, reducing waste, and using value stream maps to improve understanding and throughput. Six Sigma uses teams that are assigned well-defined projects that have direct impact on the organization's bottom line. All levels receive training in statistical thinking and key people are provided extensive training in advanced statistics and project management. Practitioners of the Lean Six Sigma approach must participate in a series of certification levels, known as belts. Each level signifies the practitioner's knowledge, training, and expertise. A Master Black Belt coaches black belts and green belts. A Black Belt coaches project teams and leads problem-solving projects. A Green Belt helps with data collection and analysis for Black Belt projects and leads Green Belt projects. The Yellow Belt acts as a member of the project team and reviews process improvements and the white Belt works in problem-solving teams as a beginner.

Six Sigma has a defined set of tools, and both qualitative and quantitative techniques are used to drive process improvement. A few tools include statistical process control (SPC), control charts, failure mode and effects analysis, and process mapping. The methodology of Six Sigma is the approach known as DMAIC (define, measure, analyze, improve and control). DMAIC defines the steps a Six Sigma practitioner is expected to follow, starting with identifying the problem and ending with the implementation of long-lasting solutions. While DMAIC is not the only Six Sigma methodology in use, it is certainly the most widely adopted and recognized. Six Sigma quality performance means 3.4 defects per million opportunities (accounting for a 1.5-sigma shift in the mean).

DMAIC Model

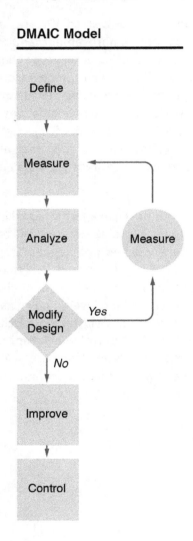

Identifying Process Champions

The term *process champion* is applied to the administrative leader who is a team member. This person should have the authority to allocate the time and resources needed to plan and launch the program. They must also have authority over the areas that will be affected by changes to clinical and administrative systems and practices; and coordinate communication internally to senior leadership, Board of Directors, staff, etc. They provide positive action-oriented leadership to ensure that process improvement projects get across the goal line.

In addition to a process champion, a clinical team may have a Primary Care Provider champion who has a vested interest in improving a clinical process. The PCP Champion may also participate in review of post-launch metrics to evaluate program success and help brainstorm solutions to areas of the program that need adjustment.

A process Improvement champion should be proficient in business and operations, project selection, pacing and results implementation. They should also have the following characteristics:

- Ability to envision, and translate it into reality (strategic intelligence)
- Culture builder by enacting values
- Alignment of business and social interests (social relevance)
- Teach others to be leaders as well
- Develop and empower trust at all levels
- Developing win-win teamwork with external partners
- Distinguishing personal ideology and values from organizational practices and strategies

Implementation and Evaluation

Establishing Teams, Roles, Responsibilities, and Scope

It is often necessary to periodically evaluate processes to eliminate waste, remove redundancies, and reduce risks, while working to expand on the gains of currently successful practices. The implementation and evaluation processes includes several key items. Key stakeholders and business leaders in healthcare organizations have an expectation of sustainable change so the best approach is to be both innovative and imaginative. Once the parameters and goals of the project have been clearly defined, defects can be rooted out and eliminated. If the tactics are successful in their implementation, the end result will help to encourage agency-specific changes aligned with the mission, goals, and values of the host organization. The team seeks out opportunities to add value to the consumer experience and improve the overall experience.

In the rapidly-changing healthcare marketplace, intermittent evaluation of the effectiveness of an organization's culture is critical. Organizational excellence cannot be built if the departments, teams, and employees are not immersed in a culture that recognizes the importance of performance improvement standards. When the staff expects to be evaluated and rewarded for adherence to performance standards, the organization can become more competitive. It is also necessary for the leadership team to model being an effective team player. This top-down approach reinforces the company culture of competence and excellence. Moving from individual to collective accountability requires significant skill. Team-building efforts must result in a cohesive team. It is crucial to qualify and quantify the effectiveness of team members, in order to emphasize the importance of a team approach to improving current policies, procedures, and processes. When employees feel that their contribution is linked to the mission, values, and goals of the host organization, they are more likely to accept responsibility for their results.

It is necessary to confirm the depth and breadth of each team member's knowledge base. Since direct management staff are typically well aware of the individual skill sets of their employees, they are frequently notified when the CPHQ professional must build a reasonable candidate pool for projects. Once assembled, the candidates are dispatched to their respective teams and the real work of team building can begin.

One particularly effective team-building technique is Bruce Tuckman's model. This model for team building focuses on forming, storming, norming, performing and adjourning. Initially, the manager will begin forming the team. The primary goal in this phase is to encourage discussion among colleagues. Team members are chosen based on the areas of expertise necessary to achieve optimal results. Together, the team members will create the framework of the PIP. Next, the manager will need to quiet and calm the storms, or the naturally-occurring conflicts between different team members' communication style. The goal of this step is to explain the stages of the process and confirm that each team member is aware of their expected contribution. Mutual trust in the team is built as each team member begins to recognize their separate and collective strengths. Norming is next. Norming is when team members come to recognize each other's strengths and resolve their differences. Members are encouraged to assume responsibility for their assigned roles. The manager acts as scaffolding, keeping the team members on task and fostering more collaboration. The next stage in Tuckman's model is defined as performing. During this phase, the manager can begin to take a less direct role and delegate activities to team members. Essentially, letting them do it by themselves builds each team member's confidence, competence, and skill set, which will cement individual accountability.

Four stages of team development

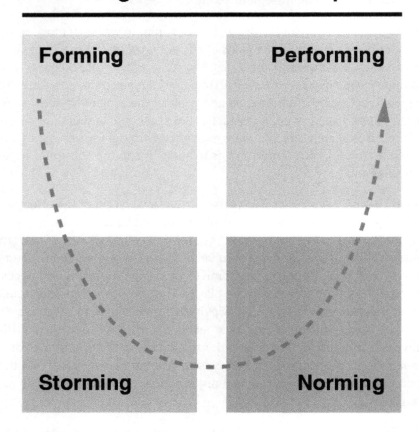

Using a Range of Quality Tools and Techniques

When creating a blueprint for current policies and procedures, it is necessary to consider the most appropriate tools for the job. Depending on the scope of the project, the size of the organization, and the goals, the project management team must use certain tools to measure a baseline and terminal success. One of the most integral tools of an effective project management team is a commitment to cooperative and collaborative teamwork. Most project management teams use tools in the early phase of the project to define the limits of the intervention. In brainstorming sessions. Each rung of the process ladder is summarized or identified. The team creates the high-level process map, adding each individual facet of the processes as needed. The map reveals which steps need improvement. The process maps are typically designed as a visual representation of the current processes, in an effort to find areas of redundancy and lack of value to the customer. This is always necessary to accomplish the goal of the project. Using clearly-labeled process maps, the team determines the basic definitions of the variables involved to accurately measure the problem.

An alternate form of program evaluation involves a more outcome-based method. Most CPHQ professionals work to determine how any given process in the system might fail. Failure mode and effect analysis (FMEA) seeks to uncover ways that business leaders can most effectively operationalize the efforts of frontline staff. The purpose is to find solutions before they become necessary. This form of program evaluation uses a qualitative approach to better understand and prevent future and ongoing threats to patient safety. The actual staff must be involved, as they can help to identify gaps in the practical application of the results. Both actual and perceived failures in practice are examined. Three questions are asked and answered: what is the severity of the effect on the customer? how often is this event likely to occur? and how easily can the customer themselves identify the problem? Each category is ranked in: potential effect; severity of the effect; potential cause and probability of occurrence; detection severity. Ranked in severity from 1 to 10 by the team, they are placed in descending order to begin the brainstorming portion of the problem-solving process. The assembled team will then begin working to create solutions to the identified problems. Wherever the actual failures are ranked as a 5 or greater, the risk assessment team will target how to implement the most effective solutions. The strategy continues with the team developing an action plan for erroneous or unnecessary steps in the current processes. As the momentum builds, more solutions become apparent.

One final format for depicting statistical data is the fishbone, or cause and effect diagram. Named precisely due to the shape, this diagram focuses largely on depicting the precipitating factors, or performing root cause analysis, for an event or outcome. Those root causes can then be separated into more meaningful categories. Practitioners can then periodically engage in the brainstorming and process mapping necessary to clarify potential solutions during each phase of the project. This format for evaluating the effectiveness of current processes is also useful achieving results aligned with the objectives and value drivers of any organization.

Participating in Monitoring of Project Timelines and Deliverables

Successful performance and process improvement requires team to participate in monitoring of the timeline and deliverable objectives. As previously mentioned, the project team needs to determine the most necessary aspects of the initiative and align them with performance metrics. When performance metrics are reviewed, the focus can shift from problem-focused to solution-focused. The apparent gaps in outcomes related to the VOC and the VOB must be addressed and the staff retrained in an effort to standardize policies, procedures, and processes. The primary goal for process improvement in program evaluation is for the team to maintain the gains achieved by identifying statistically significant processes across the organization. The value added to the customer's experience is of paramount importance. This will encourage staff adherence to new process changes, thereby ensuring continued compliance and less variation. This continuation of the define stage of the DMAIC model encourages the team to ask a series of questions as listed below. The subsequent answers will be the driving force behind all the project charter initiatives.

- Which objectives must be accomplished first?
- What are the tangible deliverables for this project?
- What is the current state?
- What is the vision for the future state?
- How frequently will progress towards the goal be evaluated?
- How, exactly, will progress towards the ultimate goal be measured?
- What is the final due date for the project?
- What are the value-added benefits to the customer?

Simply put, performance and process improvement techniques focus on delivering value to the customer.

Performance and process improvement is essentially a game of remove and replace. Antiquated or ineffective processes are removed, and they are replaced with activities designed to increase the likelihood of success. The assembled project management team must define the projected outputs, or deliverables, to be received by the customer. Next, the team must determine whether the effort of the staff to implement the new processes is outweighed by the reward delivered to consumers. The cost-benefit analysis is an activity used in the Lean Six Sigma methodology as a way to determine the true costs of a potential solution compared to the actual benefits. It is frequently necessary to conduct a cost-benefit analysis at the start of the project charter, during the define phase, and throughout implementation of the project.

While working toward creating a cohesive plan of action, the key managers and decision-makers must be well aware of the KPIs. KPIs can best be defined as measurable data that will further indicate whether the goals are attainable. These performance measures enable the team to operationalize success. When considering what may go wrong, the team must determine whether the individual actions in the newly developed processes are logical. If the steps are too complex, they may be abandoned in favor of old habits. For this reason, mistake-proofing is used, which entails developing the necessary countermeasures to solve any problems before they actually occur. Although each activity in mistake-proofing can build on the previous step, the steps are also independent. Finally, the timeliness of the resolution of the PIP is crucial. Each initiative should have a measurable timeline, but performance improvement in the organization as a whole is an ongoing commitment to excellent performance. When performance improvement projects are considered as fluid in nature, it becomes evident that the periodic evaluation of their effectiveness is mandatory.

Evaluating Team Effectiveness

It is important to note whether a team member shows up to work or not. Attendance is definitely worth tracking. If a team member consistently shows up late, leaves early, or takes an unusual number of sick days, they are not showing their full potential. Poor attendance can be caused by any number of things, including a lack of motivation, health issues, or burnout. Absenteeism can put extra pressure on other team members who have to make up for missing coworkers. Furthermore, if the organization is understaffed and team members are overworked in general, it's best to address the problem as soon as possible to avoid putting team health and well-being at risk.

Team members need to be able to complete their work on time. They should have a good handle on the limitations provided by the time and resources available and should be able to prioritize to get things done as efficiently as possible. Looking at team members who take initiative is also important for growing businesses. Rapidly changing workplaces require people who can adapt and be proactive. Initiative-taking is a difficult metric to measure, but a good place to start would be by keeping track of the times a team member takes initiative. The quality of work the team members put out is the most important metric, but it is also the most difficult to define. Team members who care about what they do and are engaged at work will likely perform better. Achievements should be recognized.

Evaluating the Success of Performance Improvement Projects

A strong commitment to improving processes and employee performance improves the organization's ability to compete in the healthcare marketplace. Evaluating the success of performance improvement measures is integral to the maintenance of project management. Best practices of performance improvement include a willingness to seek a better understanding of the VOC, or voice of the patient, as well as the VOB. It is the critical examination of the answers to these questions that will guide the expansion of the process improvement implementation from general to specific goals and change the level of difficulty for measuring the effectiveness of the interventions from problematic to less challenging. It will always be more advantageous to consider the importance of adding, rather than detracting, from the value delivered to customers.

Developed by Everett Rogers in 1962, the theory of the diffusion of innovation tries to explain how ideas and technology spread over time. Innovation is the action or process of developing a new idea, methodology, or action that improves on its predecessor. As it applies to performance improvement, diffusion can be defined as the passive and unplanned spread of new practices. This diffusion is said to occur through a five step decision-making process containing the following steps: knowledge, persuasion, decision, implementation, and confirmation.

- Knowledge: when the individual is exposed to a new idea but lacks information about the new idea.

- Persuasion: the individual becomes interested in the new idea and pursues information about it.

- Decision: the individual weighs the advantages/disadvantages and a decision is made about whether or not to accept the new idea.

- Implementation: the individual uses the new idea during this stage and determines its usefulness.

- Confirmation: the individual decides whether or not to continue using the new idea.

Effective performance improvement techniques involve training all groups in the organization. Managers must always remain diligent and remain aware that the responses of the process innovators, early adopters, and the early majority will most likely determine the success of the newly developed process and performance expectation. Once it has been determined which of the newly developed process modifications have been adopted, and to what degree, it will be necessary to determine their success.

The most necessary step in evaluating the success of process improvement is the execution of the pilot study. Participants in the pilot study need to be polled regarding their overall experience with the processes, the software, and any unexpected outcomes. It is crucial to engage with the members of the team, both individually and as a group. Which participants were responsible for encouraging other team members to endorse, adopt, and execute the process changes? Who are the process champions? How long did it take to integrate the changes in with current procedures? What, specifically, did the innovators perceive to be most effective? In what ways did the proposed process changes fail? During the improve phase of the DMAIC model, the goal is to assimilate all the ideas into a strategic plan that prioritizes opportunities for improvement. Additionally, the goal is to amend all processes associated with changes, including any process flows and job aids. Questions must be asked and answered in order for the team to adequately determine the most logical steps to document the agreed-upon process changes and improvements.

Documenting Performance and Process Improvement Results

The ultimate goal for the team professional is to empower the organization's leadership to improve their employees' performance. Strategies that are no longer effective in bringing out the best in their employees must be replaced. Performance improvement planning also requires the team to collaborate with the leadership team and guide the development of a multidimensional approach that capitalizes on the internal strengths of the organization and minimizes weaknesses. During the control phase of the DMAIC model, the team needs to implement strategies to determine the sustainability and benefits of the newly defined processes. The team looks for feasible answers to the questions asked in the improve phase.

Monitoring and reviewing the process improvement project consists of assembling the team to review all the findings associated with the pilot study and the subsequent brainstorming sessions. Lessons learned through the streamlining the ill-fitting portions of the new process will be applied. The project manager must periodically assess whether the team is on task, and it is also crucial to collect the lessons learned during each phase. This is most effective during the break-out brainstorming sessions, and once the managers have been trained on the newly developed processes.

The evaluation team will also return to review the issue logs and initiate thought process mapping, to further eliminate wasteful steps. How will gains be maintained? Have periodic process audits been established to assess the use and effectiveness of the solutions to ensure that staff do not revert to previous activities? In what ways have the results been leveraged to prevent occurrences of similar issues in all departments impacted by the problem? What is the most effective display of the findings? In an effort to prevent a recurrence of previously identified defects, the team must verify that the outcome of their action plan is functional, and they must further validate that the outcomes are aligned with the predetermined targets. Verification refers to testing that the proposed solution produces the desired outcome, while validation is a process that ensures that the outcome actually solves the problem. Once the results of the initial project are confirmed, a new project is identified, and the process begins again with the next identified issue of the organization.

The team must maintain an awareness of the nature of performance and process improvement. The goal is to train the leadership teams on the best practices to conduct performance and process improvement reviews periodically, utilizing the most effective methods. Once proficient in the Lean Six Sigma methodology, trained leaders become trainers themselves. The professional accountability and adherence to ongoing performance and process improvement measures afford the chosen organization the opportunity to remain competitive in the healthcare marketplace.

Practice Questions

1. What is the best definition for critical to quality measures (CTQs)?
    a. The correlation, or dependent relationship between two quantitative continuous variables, whether positive or negative
    b. The necessary countermeasures to solve any problems before they actually occur
    c. The measurable data that will further indicate whether the goals and objectives are attainable
    d. The aspects of a business process or product that must be met in order to satisfy the consumer

2. Before sending out a meeting invite, what is the most important thing the facilitator must do?
    a. decide who to have on the team
    b. get approval from administration
    c. define the objective of the meeting
    d. set goals

3. What is the major advantage of using scorecards and dashboards during a process and performance improvement?
    a. Both are designed as a visual representation of the current processes, in an effort to find areas of redundancy and lacking in value to the customer.
    b. Using scorecards and dashboards during a performance review can help highlight areas where additional training around related processes and procedures is needed.
    c. The election and introduction of team members based on the areas of expertise helps to achieve optimal results.
    d. Both individual and collective contributions of employees are recognized, reinforcing the establishment of the newly developed skills.

4. What is work performance data?
    a. A written document designed to be a visual roadmap for process improvement
    b. Measurable data that indicates whether the goals and objectives are attainable
    c. Raw data related to the occurrence of specific task.
    d. The dependent relationship between two quantitative continuous variables, either positive or negative.

5. What is the best definition for brainstorming?
    a. The action or process of developing a new idea, methodology, or action that improves on its predecessor
    b. The provider of inputs into a process
    c. Using a selected group of individuals to rapidly produce, clarify, and evaluate ideas or problems
    d. The way to determine the true costs of a potential solution compared to the actual benefits

6. What is the purpose of the dashboard in performance improvement?
    a. Dashboards are tools that enable the management team to visually analyze the KPIs of each individual on the healthcare team.
    b. Dashboards depict the precipitating factors or root cause for an event or outcome
    c. Dashboards contain measurable data that indicates whether the goals and objectives are attainable.
    d. Dashboards are a written account that compares and measures the performance of individuals against the projected goals of the organization.

7. How frequently are scorecards used internally for performance improvement?
   a. Quarterly
   b. Quarterly and annually
   c. Annually
   d. Monthly

8. What is the purpose of the cost-benefit analysis in process improvement?
   a. To determine the true costs of a potential solution compared to the actual benefits
   b. To ensure that the outcome actually solves the problem
   c. To confirm the passive and unplanned spread of new practices
   d. To find solutions before they become necessary

9. What is the advantage of identifying process champions for process and performance improvement projects?
   a. Process champions provide a visual representation of the current processes, in an effort to find areas of redundancy and lacking in value to the customer.
   b. It will always be more advantageous to consider the importance of adding to, rather than detracting from, the value delivered to customers.
   c. Process champions includes can identify potential pitfalls during the brainstorming phase of process improvement.
   d. Process champions ensure that the VOC is heard and to confirm that there is a precisely defined focus on the correct processes.

10. The core portions of the SIPOC method include which of the following?
    a. Suppliers, inputs, processes, outputs, customers
    b. Scorecards, inputs, processes, outputs, customers
    c. Sponsors, investors, products, outputs, customers
    d. Suppliers, inputs, processes, opportunities, consumers

11. What is the goal of the improve phase of the DMAIC model?
    a. To enable the management team to visually analyze the KPIs of each individual on the healthcare team
    b. To assimilate all the ideas into a strategic plan that prioritizes opportunities for improvement and amends all processes associated with changes, including any process flows and job aids
    c. During the improve phase of the DMAIC model, the CPHQ professional will need to implement strategies to determine the sustainability and benefits of the newly defined processes.
    d. During this phase, the manager enables team members to do it themselves.

12. Broken down into each individual function, what does the acronym DMAIC stands for?
    a. Define, measure, analyze, improve, control
    b. Define, measure, adjust, improve, complete
    c. Define, measure, amend, institute, control
    d. Depict, measure, analyze, improve, control

13. What does the project charter typically include?
   a. The sponsor or the project, a champion or resource allocation manager, subject matter expert, process owner, process operator
   b. The primary reason for the project, the goal, the scope of the project, the budget and roles of each team member
   c. Yellow belt, green belt, black belt, master black belt, process champion, executives.
   d. Suppliers of inputs, materials to input, processes that convert inputs to outputs, outputs to provide to customers, customers

14. Why is it important to review scorecards and dashboards during performance improvement projects?
   a. The professional accountability and adherence to ongoing performance and process improvement measures afford the chosen organization the opportunity to remain competitive in the healthcare marketplace.
   b. Managers must always remain diligent and keenly aware that the responses of the process innovators, early adopters, and the early majority will most likely determine the success of the newly developed process and performance expectation.
   c. The results from the aggregated quality and performance data equip the management team to develop specific, measurable, achievable, relevant, and timely (SMART) metrics for gauging the staff's effectiveness and efficiency.
   d. When employees feel that their contribution is linked to the mission, values, and goals of the host organization, they are more likely to accept responsibility for their results.

15. A facilitator needs to consider all EXCEPT which of the following?
   a. The time available for meetings
   b. The structure of the meeting
   c. Which goals to set
   d. The number of team members

16. Why is it crucial to consider the voice of the customer (VOC) during process improvement?
   a. The customer's voice is the outward image of the business, and the reputation that the business has earned among consumers.
   b. The voice of the customer uses a selected group of individuals to rapidly produce, clarify, and evaluate ideas or problems.
   c. The customer's voice enables the leadership team to understand the passive and unplanned spread of new practices.
   d. During this phase, the manager can begin to take a less direct role and delegate activities to team members.

17. Why should correlations be reviewed with caution during process and performance improvement projects?

    a. At this stage, it is crucial to create linkages between the mission, goals, and objectives of the host organization to the actual performance metrics, skills, and quality standards of the supportive team members.

    b. The CPHQ professional will need to implement strategies to determine the sustainability and benefits of the newly defined processes.

    c. When considering what may go wrong, the team professional must determine whether the individual actions in the newly developed processes are logical.

    d. The team must remain aware that the data may only represent the relationship between variables, not the actual causes and effects of current processes.

18. A team meeting is considered successful only if:

    a. actions have follow-up

    b. there are clear activities

    c. process owners are present

    d. all of the above

19. Which of the following is true regarding Critical to Quality measures?

    a. They are defined by the leadership team

    b. They are set by CMS

    c. They must be met to satisfy the customer

    d. They are always key processes

20. What happens when the needs of the business do not meet the needs of the customer?

    a. Resources are exhausted

    b. Processes have failed

    c. Voice of the customer is needed

    d. Certification is not possible

21. What is the order of the Lean Six Sigma certification belts according to rising expertise level?

    a. Yellow, green, black, master black

    b. Black, yellow, green, master black

    c. Master black, green, yellow, black

    d. Green, yellow, black, master black

22. The action plan should include which of the following?

    a. Missing capacities

    b. Signatures of all team members

    c. Who, what, when, where, why and how

    d. A way to track progress

23. Output is:

    a. tangible results

    b. goods and services

    c. under team control

    d. all of the above

24. Indicators are:
    a. linked to objectives
    b. measurable
    c. linked to quality
    d. all of the above

25. When does implementation occur?
    a. When the board members sign off on the project
    b. When everyone on the team agrees on the process
    c. When practices are adopted and integrated
    d. When the team finishes its work

26. Which of the following is included in the PLAN stage of PDSA?
    a. Complete the action plan
    b. Develop the calendar
    c. Test the validity of the plan
    d. Identify possible interventions

27. Lean Six Sigma drives customer satisfaction and the bottom line by doing which of the following?
    a. Analyzing PDSA steps closely
    b. Using Pareto charts to track improvement
    c. Using competitive benchmarking
    d. Reducing variation and waste

28. What is the BEST definition for key performance indicators (KPIs)?
    a. The provider of inputs into a business process
    b. Measurable data that indicates whether the goals and objectives are attainable
    c. Materials and resources needed to complete a business process
    d. The products or services resulting from inputs during the implementation of a process

29. What is the BEST definition for mistake-proofing?
    a. Finding ways to determine whether there is a dependent relationship between two quantitative continuous variables, can either be positive or negative
    b. Using a selected group of individuals to rapidly produce, *clarify,* and *evaluate* ideas or problems
    c. Developing the necessary countermeasures to solve any problems before they actually occur
    d. The election and introduction team members based on the areas of expertise necessary to achieve optimal results

30. What is the BEST definition of cost-benefit analysis?
    a. Testing that the proposed solution produces the desired outcome
    b. Quality measurement tools that actually enable the management team to visually analyze the KPIs of each individual on the healthcare team
    c. The action or process of developing a new idea, methodology or action, that improves on its predecessor
    d. An activity used in the Lean Six Sigma methodology as a way to determine the true costs of a potential solution compared to the actual benefits

31. What is the BEST definition of norming?
    a. Norming is when people begin to resolve their differences and come to accept their coworkers' strengths.
    b. Norming is a process that ensures that the outcome actually solves the problem.
    c. Norming is the passive and unplanned spread of new practices.
    d. Norming is measurable data that will further indicate whether the goals and objectives are attainable.

32. What is the BEST description for the purpose of storming?
    a. To develop countermeasures to solve any problems before they actually occur
    b. To explain the stages of the process and confirm that each team member is aware of their expected contribution
    c. To adopt and integrate practices in the proposed setting
    d. To visually analyze the KPIs of each individual on the healthcare team

33. With Tuckman's model (forming, storming, norming, performing) what is the primary goal?
    a. To encourage discussion among colleagues
    b. To form a strong team
    c. To meet the goals of the organization
    d. For the team to follow the facilitator's plan

34. What is diffusion?
    a. A method of brainstorming
    b. A way to control a team that is off course
    c. The passive spread of a new process
    d. Prohibited by most organizations

35. What is the most necessary step in evaluating the success of process improvement?
    a. Teamwork
    b. Executing the pilot study
    c. Informing administration of the plans
    d. An action plan

36. Why should processes be evaluated frequently?
    a. To eliminate waste and reduce risk
    b. Because it is mandated by the Joint Commission
    c. To reinforce employee trainings
    d. To determine if they still work

37. What is a process champion?
    a. An administrative team member
    b. Someone that has authority over the involved process
    c. A member of the process improvement team
    d. All of the above

38. What is VOB?
    a. An important process measure
    b. The needs of the business owner
    c. Business-centered goals
    d. All of the above

39. What is the BEST definition of verification?
    a. The active spread of those new practices to a target audience utilizing planned methodologies
    b. A process that ensures that the outcome actually solves the problem.
    c. The testing that the proposed solution produces the desired outcome.
    d. Measurable data that will further indicate whether the goals and objectives are attainable.

40. What is the BEST definition of validation?
    a. The rate at which newly disseminated innovations are adopted and implemented
    b. Developing the necessary countermeasures to solve any problems before they actually occur
    c. A dependent relationship between two quantitative continuous variables
    d. A process that ensures that the outcome actually solves the problem

Answer Explanations

1. D: Critical to quality measures (CTQs) are the aspects of a business process or product that must be met in order to satisfy the consumer. This leads to a discovery of the voice of the customer (VOC), which is also crucial to improving processes.

2. C: Before sending out a meeting invite, the most important thing is that the facilitator must define the objectives of the meeting. They should also establish the tangible outcomes or outputs that the team aims to achieve. Doing so sets expectations and will ensure that people know precisely what is expected.

3. C: Using scorecards and dashboards during a performance review can help highlight areas where additional training around related processes and procedures is needed.

4. C: Raw performance data is taken directly from the occurrence of tasks in the process flow.

5. A: Brainstorming is the action or process of developing a new idea, methodology, or action that improves on its predecessor.

6. A: Dashboards are quality measurement tools that enable the management team to visually analyze the KPIs of each individual on the healthcare team.

7. B: Scorecards are used internally during quarterly and annual employee evaluations.

8. A: This is an activity used in the Lean Six Sigma methodology as a way to determine the true costs of a potential solution, as compared to the actual benefits.

9. C: Process champions includes can identify potential pitfalls during the brainstorming phase of process improvement.

10. A: SIPOC stands for suppliers, inputs, processes, outputs, and customers.

11. B: The goal is to assimilate all the ideas into a strategic plan that prioritizes opportunities for improvement and amends all processes associated with changes, including any process flows and job aids.

12. A: Define, measure, analyze, improve, control.

13. B: The project charter includes the primary reason for the project, the goal, the scope of the project, the budget, and the roles of each team member.

14. C: The results from the aggregated quality and performance data equip the management team to develop specific, measurable, achievable, relevant, and timely (SMART) metrics for gauging the staff's effectiveness and efficiency.

15. C: Goals are set by the team, not the facilitator.

16. A: The customer's voice is the outward image of the business, and the reputation that the business has earned among consumers.

17. D: The team must remain aware that the data may only represent the relationship between variables, not the actual causes and effects of current processes.

18. D: For a team meeting to be successful, actions must have follow-up, there must be clear activities, and process owners must be present.

19. C: Critical to Quality measures are the aspects of a business process or product that must be met in order to satisfy the consumer.

20. A: When the needs of the business do not meet the needs of the customer, resources will be exhausted.

21. A: The correct level-by-level categorization of Lean Six Sigma certification is yellow, green, black, and Master black.

22. C: The Action Plan should always include the who, what, when, where, why and how.

23. D: The outcome and outputs for each objective of an Action Plan have to be identified. While the outcome is the development outcome at the end of the NSDS implementation, or—more specifically—the expected benefits to the target groups, the outputs are the direct and tangible results (goods and services) that will be delivered. Outputs are largely under the project management control.

24. D: Indicators are linked to objectives and quality and are measurable.

25. C: Implementation occurs when practices are adopted and integrated.

26. D: The PLAN stage of the PDSA involves identifying a goal or purpose, formulating an intervention or theory for change, defining success metrics and putting a plan into action. When using PDSA to improve a process, the first step is to Identify possible goals and strategies to implement. After the goal is set, it's necessary to identify possible interventions and select one that seems promising.

27. D: Lean Six Sigma drives customer satisfaction and the bottom line by reducing variables and waste.

28. B: Key performance indicators (KPIs) are the measurable data that indicate whether the goals and objectives are attainable.

29. C: Mistake-proofing develops countermeasures to solve problems before they occur.

30. D: The cost-benefit analysis is an activity used in the Lean Six Sigma methodology as a way to determine the true costs of a potential solution compared to the actual benefits.

31. A: Norming is when people begin to resolve their differences and come to accept their coworkers' strengths.

32. B: The goal of storming is to explain the stages of the process and confirm that each team member is aware of their expected contribution.

33. A: The goal of Tuckman's model (forming, storming, norming, performing) to encourage discussion among colleagues.

34. C: Diffusion is the passive and unplanned spread of new practices.

35. B: The most necessary step in evaluating the success of process improvement is executing the pilot study.

36. A: Processes be evaluated frequently to eliminate waste and reduce risk.

37. D: A process champion is an administrative leader who is a team member with the authority to allocate the time and resources needed to plan and launch the program. The process champion should also have authority over the areas that will be affected by changes to clinical and administrative systems and practices; and coordinate communication internally to senior leadership, Board of Directors, staff, etc. They provide positive action-oriented leadership to ensure that process improvement projects get across the goal line.

38. B: The voice of the business (VOB) includes the implicit and explicit needs and requirements of the business, such as profit, competitive edge, and growth. It is an important process measure.

39. C: Verification refers to testing that the proposed solution produces the desired outcome.

40. D: Validation is a process that ensures that the outcome.

Patient Safety

Assessment and Planning

Assessing the Organization's Culture of Safety

Effective program evaluation begins with an in-depth assessment of all aspects associated with the safety of the organization. The role of a healthcare quality professional is the evaluation and ongoing review of the quality of patient safety within healthcare settings. A focus on safety is not merely the avoidance of errors. Patient safety has to be considered in every aspect of care. The healthcare quality professional confirms which policies and procedures are practical, which are outdated or ineffective, and which need to be revised.

The primary goal of patient safety is the prevention of harm through the methodical analysis of previously harmful events. This is accomplished through the systematic review of those policies and procedures both directly and indirectly related to patient safety. For example, when evaluating the provision of bedside care in a hospital setting, it is essential to assess the official and unofficial procedures of the nursing staff. This can be accomplished through shadowing randomly selected nurses and healthcare providers on multiple shifts, medical record reviews, and incident reports. Is the patient handoff conducted at the bedside, or does it frequently occur at the nurse's station? Do nurses scan the patient's wristband with each scheduled administration of medications? It is also important to ensure this culture of safety is apparent not only to clinical staff, but also to ancillary providers and the patients themselves.

Initially, the healthcare quality professional examines the organization's core mission and values. One of the most influential aspects of promoting a culture of patient safety is to assess the attitude exhibited by organizational leadership. It is the leadership team that will ultimately develop the core culture. The primary goal of this portion of the assessment is to determine if the organizational culture is an accurate reflection of the initial vision of the organization. How clearly are the core values articulated to the staff? Do the policies and procedures reflect the proposed core mission and values? How does the leadership team respond to incidents that contradict the organization's core mission and values? What actions have been taken to perform periodic internal evaluations of the staff? Healthcare quality analysists must ascertain if an actual culture of safety exists within the organization and how visible it is to patients and staff. The next step is to ensure that the culture is reinforced and find ways to enhance it.

Policies and procedures enacted by healthcare organizations to ensure patient safety typically include factors that meet The Joint Commission National Patient Safety goals. The Joint Commission established the National Patient Safety (NPS) goals in 2002 and implemented them the following year. This nationwide effort instituted a set of uniform, realistic, and specific goals that could be consistently applied and measured in every healthcare setting. National Patient Safety goals have set the standard for excellence and are set annually. Several of the most important goals applicable in every healthcare setting include: identifying patients correctly, using medications safely, preventing infection, identifying patient safety risks, and improving staff communications. Each goal requires that the leadership create an atmosphere of patient-centered care, with a focus on the interdepartmental teamwork necessary to maintain the safety of the entire patient population. Any breech in patient security should be noted, along with recommendations on the necessary adjustments. Accreditation assumes that every healthcare agency seeking recognition is interested in developing the types of programs, policies, and procedures that focus on evidence-based, clinically appropriate care. Physicians, nurses, and other healthcare providers view the accreditation of an institution as a sign of excellence. Other benefits can include the fact that many local and state governments reward healthcare organizations for being recognized through expedited licensure, waivers through Medicare and Medicaid, third-party reimbursement, and improved access to more lucrative managed care contracts.

Determining How Technology Can Enhance the Patient Safety Program

Medical records were not kept and maintained until the early 1920s, when physicians realized the importance of a patient's medical history when providing care. This practice was helpful, but patient histories were often incomplete and rarely accessible by other healthcare providers. Simply storing the numerous documents required entire rooms and often whole floors of hospitals and offices. It wasn't until the late 1960s when the first computer was created that the healthcare sector began to consider the widespread use of computers. Since the earliest computers were cumbersome and expensive, their use was common only in large hospitals and government agencies. The 1970s ushered in a need for more extensive medical record keeping. With the influx of American veterans returning home and needing significant medical and psychiatric care, paper medical files were largely traded in for computerized records. The introduction of President Obama's American Recovery and Reinvestment Act of 2009 required at least 70% of all healthcare organizations transition to electronic medical records by 2014.

The electronic health record, or EHR, is one of the primary tools utilized in the maintenance of patient safety. Within many healthcare settings, the EHR is easily accessible to physicians, pharmacists, nurses, and other ancillary providers. This allows for each individual involved in caring for a specific patient to be immediately aware of any changes in diagnoses, medications, allergies, and treatments. Medications entered hastily are flagged when contradictory information, such as other medications or allergies, is noted by the sophisticated medical software. The majority of larger medical facilities have further incorporated bedside charting for all providers so that information can be easily updated in the patient's room, and wristbands are scanned prior to medication administration to confirm that appropriate medications are dispensed.

One pitfall of the electronic medical record involves the human factor. Since a computer is only capable of providing information based on what is entered, information entered inaccurately or omitted has the potential to harm a patient. Consider a patient who enters an emergency room with an acute allergic reaction to a new medication. If the hospital is not a part of the healthcare system that the patient typically frequents, this information may not be readily available in the electronic record. This opens the door for inaccurate patient records and the possibility of harm to the patient. For these reasons, numerous companies have software specifically developed to safeguard electronic medical records. Currently, those safeguards often include extensive firewalls, applications that require rolling and random password changes, multiple tiers of medical record access, and closed network connections.

Additional technological security measures that have been instituted in healthcare organizations include those created for infants and patients managing mental health concerns. The majority of labor and delivery, nursery, and mother-baby units within hospitals are equipped with technologically enhanced abduction protocols. When admitted to the labor and delivery unit, expectant mothers receive a regular hospital wristband with a patient identification number. Once the infant is born, they also receive a similar ankle bracelet with the corresponding mother's name and his/her own patient identification number; this number is also connected with the medical records of the birth mother. Infants must travel in a bassinette and are always accompanied by medical personnel from their respective units in the hospital. Once reunited with the birth mother, both arm bands are scanned, to confirm that both the mother and child are related through the patient identification numbers. The ankle bracelet is also equipped with an alarm that will sound and disable all points of egress from the unit, to prevent abduction. A similar alert wristband is used for inpatient mental health units, those admitted from correctional facilities, or those at risk for suicide. Patients at risk for elopement are prevented from exiting the floor or entering elevators. Other rooms are equipped with cameras that continually monitor patients. Overall, the technological improvements and changes are necessary to guard the protected health information of all patients.

Participating in Risk Management Assessment Activities

It is essential to maintain strict guidelines regarding quality and patient safety. Patient safety specialists often need to collaborate with the risk management team, quality department, patient advocates, infection prevention, and members of the board of ethics. Quality professionals must have an intimate knowledge of healthcare organizations and accreditation standards, and possess the ability to apply them. The Joint Commission of Healthcare Organizations was officially formed in 1951 as a formalized and structured way to monitor patient safety in healthcare settings. Currently, The Joint Commission accredits, or recognizes, over 20,000 hospitals, nursing homes, and other healthcare organizations on the quality of care that they provide. The overall mission of this nonprofit association is to independently examine the policies and procedures that threaten patient safety, and it has become the gold standard of evidence-based medical care.

Risk management professionals employ multiple tactics to evaluate patient safety in healthcare organizations. The three main principles of risk management assessment are risk assessment, risk avoidance, and risk control. Risk assessment is the initial and most important step in the process. What happened and why? The analyst will need access to all available records, participants, policies, and procedures associated with the event. Methodical and purposeful deconstruction of every step should be mapped, and any discrepancies in processes, hardware, human factors, and organizational culture scrutinized. Similar incidents and associated resolutions within other healthcare settings should be compared and analyzed for probability of success. The avoidance of future risk forms the foundation for the next step: the analyst's review of the plan for potential vulnerabilities. What specific actions, policies, and procedures would prevent this type of incident in the future? What safeguards need to be in place at various stages in related procedures to undergird current processes? Finally, the risk management team develops measures to increase quality of care through the adaptation of specific control measures.

The following example highlights the application of this strategy:

A patient admitted for a below-the-knee amputation of the left leg reported a concern to the nursing manager. According to the patient, the physician entered the room, discussed the procedure, and marked the right leg for the procedure. When the patient protested, the physician advised him that the medical chart indicated the right leg as the limb to be removed. When the patient continued to protest and refused to sign the consent form for the incorrect limb, the physician cancelled the surgery and left the room angrily. When the nursing manager reviewed additional patient records, it was revealed that the patient had been correct; somehow, the medical record had been updated incorrectly the previous evening. The patient had developed a decubitus ulceration on the right heel, which was scheduled for debridement. The physician that reviewed the notes assumed that the right limb, not the left, would be removed. The nurse manager consulted the physician, and the surgery was rescheduled for the correct limb. A risk management team was assembled to review this near-miss event and it became clear that there was a miscommunication during the patient handoff from the surgical resident to the attending surgeon.

Two issues were noted during the risk assessment: The policy to conduct patient report at the bedside was not followed, and the correct limb was not marked per NPS guidelines. This incident could be avoided in the future by following established procedures regarding surgery time out. To control the likelihood of this event being repeated, the quality professional proposed that the surgical team receive additional training regarding the time-out requirements and procedures regarding bedside report. Continued education credits were provided to clinical staff as part of their annual continuing education requirements. Finally, the leadership team released a facility-wide newsletter, which included a brief synopsis of the event and the NPS guidelines regarding bedside report and surgery time out. The next step is to facilitate ongoing adherence to new patient safety guidelines.

Implementation and Evaluation

Facilitating the Ongoing Evaluation of Safety Activities

One of the most significant and effective practices that healthcare quality professionals can employ in risk assessment is the Lean Six Sigma method. Although initially developed in the manufacturing sector, the Lean Six Sigma method of assessing and managing risk has taken root in healthcare. Lean Six Sigma experts strive to reach 99.99966% of the expected goal of the is the patient. Any deviation from the standard processes typically results in higher risks to the patient. The basic principles of Lean Six Sigma in relation to the management of decreasing risks to patient safety include:

- Define the expected outcome
- Measure the actual versus perceived risk
- Analyze the scope of the risk to patients
- Improve the typical versus the most-desirable outcomes
- Control the ongoing risks to patients

When improvement is required for existing processes, Lean Six Sigma helps to define, measure, analyze, improve, and control quality—or DMAIC—with staff empowered to collect the data. For process improvement that requires significant procedural changes. The DMAIC model allows for the methodical development of an action plan to streamline and standardize laborious processes, reduce waste, and mitigate risks to the patient population in any healthcare setting. One additional outflow in this process is to consider the Lean 5S method: sort, simplify, sweep, standardize, self-discipline. The priority for this facet of Lean Six Sigma is to teach the leadership team the importance of improving simplification. This exercise encourages managers and executives to model ways to remove all nonessential items in their work environment. The exercise informs their understanding of the adjustments required of front-line staff. All are emboldened to offer strategies that remove redundant processes, while increasing the focus on what the is vital.

In the initial step, Lean Six Sigma professionals partner with the leadership of healthcare organizations and their risk management team to create an assessment of current processes. The team then works to create a process map, formulate problem and goal statements, and identify the specific needs of patients and medical staff. This approach is solution focused, and unidirectional. Each interdepartmental connection is assessed for interruptions in current processes. Raw quantitative data, in the form of near-miss and sentinel events, are gathered and analyzed. Incident reports are also reviewed in an effort to backtrack and pinpoint any breakdowns in processes, areas for improving the skillset of each employee, and ways to increase the quality of care provided. Process maps are compared with actual staff activities and then restructured around the new, more practical solutions. Finally, the team will work with leadership to ensure that the new response plan is effective and discuss methods to integrate new processes throughout the organization.

Integrating Safety Concepts Throughout the Organization

Upon completion of the analysis of any near-miss or sentinel event, the findings must be integrated into the current policies and procedures. Controlling the incidence and prevalence of sentinel events involves implementing practices that also improve the quality of care provided to patients. Technological advances in medical care have dramatically impacted healthcare delivery and overall patient safety. From the EHR to abduction and elopement security systems to smart medication pumps, innovations can either enhance or endanger overall patient safety. Proponents of patient safety often speak to the benefits of utilizing technology to augment current processes. Accurate record keeping allows quality specialists to protect the interests of the organization and the patient. Tracking the incidence and prevalence of near-miss and sentinel events is vital to meeting local and governmental regulations. The leadership team is responsible for organizing, coordinating, and facilitating the development of programs that control the clinical risks associated with patient care services in healthcare organizations. The organization must periodically conduct utilization reviews to uncover documentation irregularities. Most often, safety audits begin with reviews of patient medical records; this necessitates the importance of the standardization of documentation in the legal medical records.

Patient safety has become synonymous with risk management. Unfortunately, despite the numerous safeguards, individuals evaluating the level of care that patients receive must develop practices that confront those risks. Quality control specialists require extensive knowledge in the management of patient relations and how to de-escalate conflict. Communication skills, team building, and leadership effectiveness are all integral to the maintenance of established patient safety goals.

Risk management agents work diligently to ensure that the medical treatments patients receive do not result in associated risks. They are trained to evaluate the potential for harm as well as the causes for real events. They act when near-miss or sentinel events occur and periodically review national statistics in an effort to prevent future incidents. Whenever a healthcare provider engages in activities that contradict the current policies and procedures of the organization, those actions can and often do result in actual or potential harm to the patient. Emphasis remains on how to design and alter work processes to focus on safety, quality, and improved performance standards for the hospital system. The ultimate goal of the integration of risk management and quality control in healthcare program evaluation is to streamline current processes in favor of more efficient and effective methods.

Using Safety Principles

Professionals that examine the principles of patient safety and quality management use qualitative and quantitative data to measure the impact of errors in healthcare delivery. Qualitative research in risk management yields data in the form of concepts, which gives insight and understanding to contributing factors. Quantitative investigation reveals raw numbers, which are then typically translated into more familiar and relatable terms. The EHR forced facilities to install costly software with no guarantee that it would meet their needs. Numerous firewalls and passwords cannot always prevent basic human error when data are entered. High-reliability organizations often flourish in adversity with above-average security measures. Proponents of systems analysis combine the deeper dive with a broad view and tie all of the factors together. Critical analysis of each element within the system facilitates improved functioning of the organization as a whole. Each form of data is combined to further the goal of increasing patient safety.

It is important to consider the ethical and financial cost of breaches in patient safety. Adverse events within healthcare organizations results in a loss of credibility for a particular organization, but also can be catastrophic to the entire healthcare industry. Hospitals may lose the confidence of patients and may even face excessive financial losses. Failures to address the root cause and the subsequent effects of near-miss and sentinel events profoundly affect the patients and medical staff, extended families, friends, and society. The more significant the event is, the higher the likelihood of the offending organization dissolving.

Using an ongoing team approach develops strategies for predicting and preventing the incidence of sentinel and near-miss events. Evidence-based practice has revealed that certain principles, when followed, improve overall patient safety. Although no specific method is significantly more valuable than any other; each has its own merit. The similarities of each technique can be found in the shared goals of enhancing the overall culture of safety, and the mitigation of risk to patients. Techniques such as systems thinking and introducing the methods associated with high-reliability organizations have produced significant advances in risk management.

Human-Factors Engineering
Human-factors engineering, also known as ergonomics, is a discipline that develops devices and technology based on the physical and psychological needs of those who use them. This field combines technological advances in healthcare with the specific needs of humans in mind.

As an example, the nurse manager of a thirty-bed medical surgical unit was advised of a near-miss medication error for an elderly patient receiving hypertensive medications. Although the error was caught before the patient received the medication, the director of nursing assembled a risk management team to review the case. The patient had been admitted earlier that morning, was transferred to the inpatient unit after an episode of syncope at a local skilled nursing facility, and the attending physician requested that the patient be admitted for a head computed tomography (CT) scan to determine if any head injury had occurred. The patient's diagnoses included Alzheimer's disease and hypertension. The patient was nonverbal, and no family members were available at the time of the admission. The patient was admitted with the same medication list, but the attending physician called in additional orders at the time of admission. Orders to discontinue the hypertensive medications to rule out hypotension as a cause for the fall were not transcribed or discussed during the transition of care to the next nurse. This example underscores the human factors involved in evaluating patient safety activities. Human fallibility is the cause for this near miss.

Human-factors engineering focuses on how to build technology through usability testing, forcing functions, and as a work around. Usability explains how the device is used in a real-world situation. Forcing functions prevents one step from being completed without a prior necessary step. This case presents an opportunity to enhance patient handoffs, encourage immediate order transcription, or to institute a policy adding a secondary nurse to electronically cosign medication administration at the bedside. This event also presents an opportunity for departmental leadership to offer training and discussion regarding the importance of highlighting the overall culture of quality within the department.

High Reliability
There are five specific factors that make operating as a high-reliability organization advantageous: reliance on practical experience, loyalty in adversity, an outcome-focused approach, an emphasis on

operationalized definitions of expected outcomes, and a deeper-dive perspective when unexpected problems arise. Organizations that adopt this method of risk management achieve a high level of excellence because they focus on anticipating the best response to the worst-case scenario.

The Joint Commission has established benchmarks for quality that drive the high-reliability organization to consistently anticipate probable threats to patient safety. This model also provides transparency, accountability, and shared responsibility within the organization that reinforces problem solving. It also increases facility-wide awareness of new initiatives that reinforce patient safety. Equipped with this qualitative approach to risk management, the leadership team can prepare to follow the data points where they lead. These occurrences are not desired, but they are used as opportunities.

A sentinel event involving the death of a patient in an intensive care unit, after an anaphylactic reaction to a hastily administered blood transfusion, can be examined using the standard high-reliability approach. Facilities that utilize this approach would begin with a roundtable discussion to reveal the basic facts of the incident. Critical care nurses who routinely infuse blood, as well as emergency room nurses, would serve as the practical experts in this case. The nurse in question would not be abandoned, but educated on the best practices as evidenced by the techniques of more experienced colleagues. Their collective experience can help shed light on which procedural steps were missed or how current practices may be inadequate. A more in-depth exploration of the contributing factors, and a focus on established procedures, helps to expose gaps in current processes. Once uncovered, the risk management team can begin to work quickly to find the solution.

Systems Thinking

Systems thinking involves a more holistic approach to risk management assessment. One main goal is to understand how the different parts of the whole system work together. While typical program evaluation tends to compartmentalize, this approach investigates each incident based on how the separate systems within the hospital network have influenced an outcome. This method deconstructs the incident without an expected conclusion. Systems thinking involves asking two questions. How does each separate system contribute to the problem? In what ways can each system contribute to the solution? Recognizing that each department is itself a subsystem, equally dependent on the other departments, exposes the complex relationship as it relates to the whole. It is impossible to provide excellent care to patients without the interdependency of the entire facility.

Systems thinking also enlists cognitive mapping as a way to represent physical locations. Areas where each subsystem perceives its connections to the others can help identify still more points of interaction that contributed to the sentinel event. Does each separate department have the capacity to identify and accept responsibility for their contribution to the problem? Quality experts are also assembled for the purpose of integrating departmental perspectives to identify patterns. Often, these unexpected results help to formulate a cohesive picture of how the system has broken down.

Systems thinking is also vital in building confidence throughout the organization. The ability to rely on each individual department to demand individual and collective responsibility for their own parts in the process sets the stage for interdepartmental transparency and accountability. Systems thinking challenges antiquated and inadequate processes to protect the patient population of any healthcare setting.

Participating in Safety and Risk Management Activities

Incident Report Review
The next step is to review the incident report. The nurses and other involved staff must be interviewed. Did the nurse follow every step in the established protocol? Is it possible that the nurse may have been overtired or overextended with too many patients? Staffing models should be examined to determine if the nurse-to-patient ratios are adequate for each shift. In this instance, clinical quality specialists must collaborate with clinical and administrative personnel to create a workable plan of action. Once the required information has been gathered, the next step is to present the findings for the leadership of the organization to conduct a final review and root-cause analysis.

Sentinel/Unexpected Event Review
A sentinel event is an unforeseen occurrence that results in actual harm or death to a patient or a group of patients. In Healthcare risk management, an action or inaction that may have resulted in nonlethal injury to a patient is known as a near-miss event. Once uncovered, a near-miss or sentinel incident highlights the policies and procedures that resulted in the error. Risk management assessments must also involve an examination of problematic behaviors within the organization that foster an unsafe environment. Simply updating obsolete policies or procedures cannot completely mitigate risk. It is often necessary to deconstruct hierarchies, review organizational management charts, leadership attitudes, and the overall culture of safety. Adverse events are often associated with debilitating injuries and the risk management team can employ various techniques to analyze the actual and potential causes of the events. Formal and informal nursing practices are scrutinized, as habitual behaviors can lead to complacency. Quality and patient safety professionals then evaluate the current departmental and accreditation standards. Once it is determined which areas do not meet or exceed evidence-based standards and practices, a full risk management team is assembled to establish more effective protocols.

The risk management team must consist of individuals who value the organizational structure as much as they value patient safety. Medical records, incident reports, and at least one completely objective healthcare quality professional must be involved. The review panel must also include a representative from the internal ethical review board. This will ensure an accurate appraisal of the ethical implications of the incident. It will be necessary to determine which steps in the protocol led to the near-miss or sentinel event, and at which point the risk assessment team could intervene in order to prevent a recurrence of a similar incident.

Root-Cause Analysis
Root-cause analysis is used to evaluate patient safety in healthcare organizations. The tool identifies the underlying causes of sentinel and near-miss events and helps develop safeguards to prevent the recurrence of the incidents. In a root–cause analysis, a healthcare quality evaluator asks a series of "why" questions regarding the incident. This process is implemented to sift through current policies and reveal causal factors within the control of the team. Patient factors are not included in this step. The team must be able to influence the root cause for the modifications to be successful. The analyst must determine a causal factor from a root cause. Although some events are identified through the detection of a near miss, a sentinel event, or an incident report, other causes may involve employees or patients requesting a resolution. This systemic approach does not insist solely upon individual accountability, but rather a consideration of areas of improvement within the organization.

Consider the following example regarding the analysis of a near-miss event, and how this event can be avoided in future interactions:

A patient being treated in an urgent care clinic was almost given a medication that would have caused an anaphylactic allergic reaction. Utilizing the "five why's," it was determined that there were multiple contributing factors. Several nurses were out sick with the flu, causing higher nurse-to-patient ratios; the nurse involved had a total of ten patients, which is more than double the allowable ratio of one-to-four ratio for the clinic. Although the nurse had received the appropriate orders from the attending physician regarding the medications, it was a verbal order, which the overextended nurse failed to transcribe. This led to a failure to add the new medication to the electronic medical record. The failure to adhere to the safeguard of scanning wristbands to retrieve the computerized medication was a significant breech in the quality of care. Interdepartmental breakdowns in staffing models, protocols for vaccinations of nursing staff, and policies for accepting verbal orders may have all influenced this near miss. This root-cause analysis opens the dialogue to examine the best methods to verify improvement once the new processes are implemented.

Failure Mode and Effects Analysis

An alternate form of program evaluation involves a more outcome-based method. Quality and safety professionals work to determine how any given process within the system might fail. Failure mode and effect analysis is not a quantitative approach, but does seek to uncover ways the departments can operationalize their efforts. The purpose is to find solutions before they are needed. This form of program evaluation enlists a qualitative approach to better understand and prevent future and ongoing threats to patient safety. The actual staff must be involved, as they can help identify gaps in the practical application of the results. Both actual and perceived failures in practice are examined. Three specific questions are asked and answered: What is the severity of the effect on the patient?; How often is this event likely to occur?; and, How easily can the patient independently identify the problem? Each category is ranked by potential effect, severity of the effect, the potential cause and probability of occurrence, and detection severity. Ranked in severity from 1 to 10 by the team, they are placed in descending order to begin the brainstorming portion of the problem-solving process. The assembled team then begins working to create solutions to the identified problems. Wherever the actual failures rank as a 5 or greater, the risk assessment team targets how to implement the most effective solutions. The process continues with the team developing an action plan and as momentum builds, more solutions become apparent. Quality analysts then examine the evidence within the incident report and compare the findings to similar events. Gaps in processes are filled and strengths leveraged within the system to prevent future recurrence of the event. The success of the intervention is determined by process improvement, and evidenced by a lower incidence of comparable events.

Practice Questions

1. How does a healthcare risk management assessment typically begin?
    a. Interviewing the patient to get his/her reaction.
    b. Meeting with attorneys to discuss possible causes of the incident.
    c. Reviewing the incident report.
    d. Interviewing the leadership of the organization.

2. Which of the following statements is true regarding the policies and procedures for healthcare settings?
    a. They ensure patient safety and typically include factors that meet The Joint Commission National Patient safety goals.
    b. Many focus on developing devices and technology based on the physical and psychological needs of those who use them.
    c. The purpose is to evaluate patient safety in healthcare organizations and identify the underlying causes of sentinel and near-miss events, and then develop safeguards to prevent the recurrence of the incidents.
    d. They use a quality approach to better understand and prevent future and ongoing threats to patient safety.

3. Root-cause analysis is used to do which of the following?
    a. Identify the cause of sentinel and near miss events
    b. Evaluate patient safety
    c. Answer the "why" questions
    d. All of the above

4. What does the acronym NPS refer to?
    a. New Patient Safety
    b. National Patient Safety
    c. Net Promoter Score
    d. National Population Safety

5. Which statement about near-miss and sentinel events is true?
    a. Both are ways to define an accident in a healthcare setting.
    b. Both events always prove that the provider was negligent in caring for the patient.
    c. A near-miss event does not result in death, while a sentinel event may result in death.
    d. The responsible party should always contact the police immediately.

6. Which of the following is true about FMEA?
    a. It is a program evaluation method that is primarily process based.
    b. It is a program evaluation method that is primarily outcome based.
    c. It is a program evaluation method that is primarily observation based
    d. It is a program evaluation method that is mandated by OSHA.

7. The need for more extensive medical record keeping increased during what time period?
    a. 1950s
    b. 1960s
    c. 1970s
    d. 1980s

8. The most problematic issues of the EHR are caused by which of the following?
    a. Security measures
    b. Cyber crimes
    c. Human errors
    d. Passwords

9. Extra safety and security measures are important for which specialized hospital area?
    a. ICU
    b. ED
    c. Surgery
    d. Nursery

10. Any deviation from the standard process typically results in higher risk, according to which methodology?
    a. 5 S
    b. Six Sigma
    c. Lean
    d. National Safety Standards

11. Loyalty in adversity and an outcome-focused approach are 2 of the 5 factors of which of the following?
    a. Human Factor Engineering
    b. Standard Operating Procedures
    c. Lean/Six Sigma
    d. A high reliability organization

12. Risk Managers are trained to evaluate which of the following?
    a. Potential for harm
    b. Outcomes of events
    c. Patient safety
    d. All of the above

13. Systems Thinking uses which of the following?
    a. A centrist approach
    b. Cognitive mapping
    c. Scorecards
    d. Technology to drive ideas

14. Which Lean Six Sigma format targets current processes?
    a. Define, measure, analyze, improve, and control
    b. Define, maintain, analyze, improve, and control
    c. Define, measure, analyze, design, and verify
    d. Define, measure, analyze, investigate, and contain

15. What factors are the primary focus of human-factors engineering?
    a. Devices/technology based on the physical and psychological needs of those who use them.
    b. How to build technology through asking a series of "why" questions.
    c. Reliance on practical experience, loyalty in adversity, and an outcome-focused approach.
    d. Build technology through measurement, analysis, and improving current technology.

16. In Healthcare risk management, an action or inaction that could have resulted in nonlethal injury to a patient is known as which of the following?
  a. A sentinel event
  b. An incident
  c. A near-miss event
  d. A human factor

17. Organizations that adopt which of the following methods of risk management achieve a high level of excellence because they focus on anticipating the best response to the worst-case scenario?
  a. High Reliability
  b. Six Sigma
  c. Systems Thinking
  d. Human Factor Engineering

18. Cognitive mapping is important in the systems thinking approach because it is a way to do which of the following?
  a. Visualize what happened during the incident.
  b. Visualize otherwise unnoticeable connections.
  c. Visualize what the patient was thinking.
  d. Visualize what to do next.

19. What is the purpose of the "five why's" in a root-cause analysis?
  a. To sift through current policies and reveal causal factors within the control of the team.
  b. To make sure patients understand what happened.
  c. To prepare an incident report.
  d. To communicate the cause to the leadership of the organization.

20. Which of these statements about failure mode and effect analysis is NOT true?
  a. Failure mode analysis is an outcome-based method of program evaluation.
  b. Failures are ranked in severity from one to five, and managed in order of severity of three or greater.
  c. Analysts ask about the severity, probable cause, potential for harm, and patient detection.
  d. Failure mode analysts interview the patients involved in the incident.

Answers Explanations

1. C: The incident report is reviewed first in most healthcare risk management assessments. Recall that the three main principles of risk management assessment are risk assessment, risk avoidance, and risk control. In the most critical step, risk assessment, what happened and why and why is considered. The analyst will need access to all available records, participants, policies, and procedures associated with the event. Methodical and purposeful deconstruction of every step should be mapped, and any discrepancies in processes, hardware, human factors, and organizational culture scrutinized. Similar incidents and associated resolutions within other healthcare settings should be compared and analyzed for probability of success.

2. A: The majority of policies and procedures enacted by healthcare organizations to ensure patient safety include factors that meet The Joint Commission's requirements and National Patient Safety goals.

3. D: All of the above.

4. B: NPS is the acronym for National Patient Safety. The Joint Commission established the NPI goals in 2002 and implemented them in 2003. This nationwide effort instituted a set of uniform, realistic, and specific goals that could be consistently applied and measured in every healthcare setting. National Patient Safety goals are set annually and have established the standard for excellence.

5. C: A near-miss event does not result in death, while a sentinel event may result in death.

6. B: Failure mode and effect analysis (FMEA) is a program evaluation method that is primarily outcome based. It seeks to uncover ways that business leaders can most effectively operationalize the efforts of frontline staff.

7. C: The 1970s ushered in a need for more extensive medical record keeping. With the influx of American veterans returning home needing significant medical and psychiatric care, paper medical files were largely traded in for computerized records.

8. C: One pitfall of the electronic medical record involves the human factor. Since a computer is only capable of providing information based on what is entered, information entered inaccurately or omitted has the potential to harm a patient.

9. D: Nursery. Due to the possibility of an abduction there are special safeguards in place.

10. B: According to Six Sigma, any deviation from the standard process typically results in higher risk.

11. D: Loyalty in adversity and an outcome-focused approach are 2 of the 5 factors in any high-reliability organization. The other three are reliance on practical experience, an emphasis on operationalized definitions of expected outcomes, and a deeper-dive perspective when unexpected problems arise. Organizations that adopt this method of risk management achieve a high level of excellence because they focus on anticipating the best response to the worst-case scenario.

12. D: Risk managers are trained in many things including the potential for far, outcomes of events, and patient safety.

13. B: Systems thinking uses cognitive mapping to represent physical locations.

14. A: The Lean Six Sigma format that targets current processes is define, measure, analyze, improve, and control.

15. A: Devices/technology based on the physical and psychological needs of those who use them.

16. C: In healthcare risk management, an action or inaction that could have resulted in nonlethal injury to a patient is known as a near miss event. These must be reduced and eliminated as much as possible to promote quality, safe healthcare.

17. A: Organizations that adopt the High Reliability methods of risk management achieve a high level of excellence because they focus on anticipating the best response to the worst-case scenario.

18. B: Cognitive mapping in systems thinking helps to represent physical locations. Areas where each subsystem perceives its connections to the others can help identify still more points of interaction that contributed to the sentinel event.

19. A: The "5 Why's" help sift through current policies and reveal causal factors within the control of the team.

20. B: It is not true that failures are ranked in severity from 1-5, and managed in order of severity over the rank of 3. They are ranked for 1-10, put in descending order, and those ranked at greater than 5 are managed in order of severity.

Dear CPHQ Test Taker,

We would like to start by thanking you for purchasing this study guide for your CPHQ exam. We hope that we exceeded your expectations.

Our goal in creating this study guide was to cover all of the topics that you will see on the test. We also strove to make our practice questions as similar as possible to what you will encounter on test day. With that being said, if you found something that you feel was not up to your standards, please send us an email and let us know.

We have study guides in a wide variety of fields. If you're interested in one, try searching for it on Amazon or send us an email.

Thanks Again and Happy Testing!
Product Development Team
info@studyguideteam.com

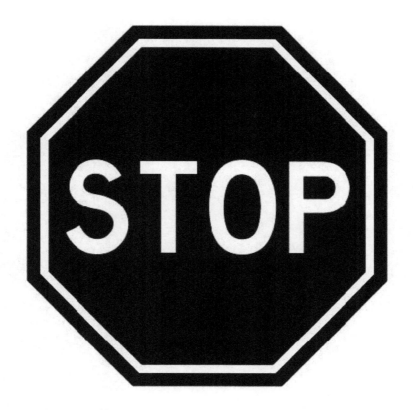

FREE Test Taking Tips DVD Offer

To help us better serve you, we have developed a Test Taking Tips DVD that we would like to give you for FREE. **This DVD covers world-class test taking tips that you can use to be even more successful when you are taking your test.**

All that we ask is that you email us your feedback about your study guide. Please let us know what you thought about it – whether that is good, bad or indifferent.

To get your **FREE Test Taking Tips DVD**, email freedvd@studyguideteam.com with "FREE DVD" in the subject line and the following information in the body of the email:

   a. The title of your study guide.

   b. Your product rating on a scale of 1-5, with 5 being the highest rating.

   c. Your feedback about the study guide. What did you think of it?

   d. Your full name and shipping address to send your free DVD.

If you have any questions or concerns, please don't hesitate to contact us at freedvd@studyguideteam.com.

Thanks again!

CPSIA information can be obtained
at www.ICGtesting.com
Printed in the USA
LVHW061947010119
602312LV00018B/1068/P